Sexual Medicine in Clinical Practice

Klaus M. Beier • Kurt K. Loewit

Sexual Medicine
in Clinical Practice

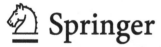 Springer

Klaus M. Beier
Institut für Sexualwissenschaft
und Sexualmedizin
Humboldt-Universität zu Berlin
Charité - Universitätsmedizin Berlin
Berlin
Germany

Kurt K. Loewit
Klinik für Medizinische
Psychologie und Psychotherapie
Universität Innsbruck
Innsbruck
Austria

ISBN 978-1-4899-8912-3   ISBN 978-1-4614-4421-3 (eBook)
DOI 10.1007/978-1-4614-4421-3
Springer New York Dordrecht Heidelberg London

Printed on acid-free paper

Springer is part of Springer Science+Business Media (www.springer.com)

Foreword

Over-viewing the past 50 years of sexual health education in the United States and Canada, the situation at medical schools, in psychology and social sciences, there is a growing body of knowledge on the one hand compared to a small amount of courses actually offered for training and often a too narrow focus on the pathological aspects of sexuality. Sexual health education needs to go deeper and broader. Unquestionably, there is a need for students and professionals alike to become skilled in the task of directly addressing their patients' sexual health concerns and enhancing their sexual functioning and well-being.

This paucity of support is all the more surprising, seeing that there is a shift from stand-alone courses and a push for more integrated learning which opens opportunities for integrating sexual health into mainstream courses. But this cannot be accomplished without a model to promote practical application for public well-being in the sense of a formalized training for medical students as well as health professionals in all fields, based on the 2002 WHO definition of sexual health "a state of physical, emotional, mental and social well-being in relation to sexuality; it is not merely the absence of disease, dysfunction or infirmity. Sexual health requires a positive and respectful approach to sexuality and sexual relationships, as well as the possibility of having pleasurable and safe sexual experiences, free of coercion, discrimination and violence."

So this book might come at just the right time. It is intended to serve as a clinical manual and addresses medical doctors and therapists first and foremost. The underlying theory of 'Syndyastics' has a much farther reaching significance and could, beyond being an effective basis for sexual therapy, promote a humanizing influence on medicine in general, on sexual health in particular and also constitute a model for preventive sex education. This is based on the fact that fundamental human needs such as the desire for acceptance, closeness and security are not only dealt with, but are seen as the vital key for the interaction between individuals over the whole life-span—from birth through old age. The focus, therefore, is on sexual health as it is experienced over the life-span concerning the quality and urgencies of life and health, and this makes it possible to use the salutogenic approach, not only in child sexual health education but also in facing the reality of ageing and increasing reliance on pharmaceutical products and medical interventions and on the impact on sexuality in terms of compromising physical and mental health with ageing in general.

This definitely corresponds with the principles of my own work and experience in group therapy and family treatment of adolescents with physical, emotional and behavioural problems, and, in particular, criminal sexual behaviour. Admittedly in a particular field, but based on the same underlying idea, our "Personal/Social Awareness Program" has corroborated the effectiveness of a holistic and sexuality-positive approach.

This supports the view on the life-span idea—as we look to understand adult sexual health on the whole—to also remember the importance of child sexual health as being the foundation of adult sexual health and to view and understand both in the context of human fundamental needs. For this reason, the Institute for Child and Adolescent Sexual Health in Minneapolis was founded in 1970s and it is distinctive for die reluctant encouragement concerning the issues in question that its maintenance has always been difficult.

With our awareness of the importance of understanding the reality of fundamental needs in nature and in the health of human beings, it is vital to also understand the importance of syndyastic sexuality in the health of children, adolescents and adults. On this basis it should be possible to initiate a major collaborative effort in the form of linked, parallel training initiatives spanning diverse field, including medicine, to cope with all the new challenges in recent times from the sex education of our children via internet to the high relevance of sexual health for an ageing population.

William Seabloom,   Institute for Advanced Study
M.Div. M.S.W. Ph.D., LICSW   in Human Sexuality,
                                                          San Francisco, CA, USA

                                                    Suite 208, Hamline Park Plaza,
                                                               570 Asbury Street,
                                                           St. Paul, MN 55104, USA

Preface

Sexual medicine touches on many aspects of primary health care. But even though some medical schools in the USA were pioneers in including courses on human sexuality in their curriculum in the 1960s and 1970s, most physicians lack formal education in the diagnosis and management of sexual and partnership-related problems, probably due to the fact that there are not enough experienced teachers in this field, meaning that educators are often uncertain how best to teach the issue lacking an evidence-based, as opposed to an individually derived, concept of human sexuality. Yet many patients seek information and advice or treatment for sexual concerns, while others hope the doctor will question them in this direction. To satisfy such demands professionally, specialized skills are called for. Although the HIV/AIDS epidemic should have been a final wake-up call to health professionals to install explicit discussion concerning sexual behaviour during routine office practice, too many physicians are still inadequately trained or prepared for dealing with sexual concerns of their patients, and/or unaware of the far reaching consequences of such disturbances for well being and health in general. During the last ten to twenty years, however, the fields of neurobiology, psychoneuroimmunology, and endocrinology have provided an impressive body of knowledge to better explain the intricate connections between health and human relations, including sexual ones, and hence to teach the issue founded on an evidence-based concept of human sexuality.

This book offers a plausible, understandable and teachable concept of sexuality ready for use in clinical practice—if the practitioner is convinced about the importance and the impact of this work, meaning that sexual health plays a significant role in life quality, that sexual and partnership problems cause both emotional and physical distress, and that sexual inquiry is an essential component of responsible and comprehensive health care.

To solve problems the right tool kit is needed, and this is true for medical health care as well. The tool kit for solving sexual and partnership problems contains resilient, evidence-based models of human attachment on the one hand and human sexual preference structure on the other. A professional who can obtain an accurate picture on this in a patient will be in a position to decode sexual disorders and develop an adequate therapy option. This tool kit is offered here, based on the authors' longstanding experience in dealing with sexual medicine in theory and practice.

Looking at an evidence-based model of human attachment, reference is made to the well-known fact that humans are phylogenetically programmed as relational beings with a social brain, disposed to pair bonding, the couple being the prime social unit. This was already perceived by the Greek philosopher Aristotle, establishing the term "syndyasticós," which serves as a template for the term "syndyastics" used in this book. Thus, the syndyastic concept comprises humans in their biopsychosocial entity as social and sexual beings seeking relationships to fulfill their fundamental needs and desires for belonging, acceptance, affection, closeness, warmth, and security, and connects these essentials of well being and health with human sexuality in its functions of bonding, lust and reproduction.

However, while everybody knows about sexual lust and reproduction, a majority of patients seeking help for sexual concerns are not conscious of the bonding, relational and hence communicative dimension of sexuality mediated to a great deal by neurobiological mechanisms such as those transmitted by Oxytocin.

During a specialized treatment (syndyastic sexual therapy) the patient(s)/couple(s) become aware of this relational and communicative function of sexuality adding a new dimension to sex and lust by connecting lust and attachment. Thus, dependent on the quality of the relationship, sexual interaction has the potential of becoming a form of non-verbal communication, mediating in a physical way belonging together, accepting each other, being close, experiencing warmth and security, in short, embodying intimacy also in the language of sexuality. Carnal and relational lust intensify each other and may lead to a new, salutogenic meaning of "sex," which no longer is unrelated or even contradictory to love.

In this context it is of utmost importance and in no way random, to determine what kind of sexual preference a person has. If, for instance, a fetishistic preference is present, this can affect sexual and partnership contentedness and cause distress during sexual interaction followed by disorders of sexual function, undermining the attachment dimension and frustrating fulfillment of the mentioned fundamental human needs.

Bearing in mind that sexual preference structure becomes manifest during puberty and remains stable for a lifetime—which is true for sexual orientation as well as for paraphilic arousal patterns—it is necessary to include this issue in the assessment in a non-judgmental way, derived from (1) knowledge about the whole range of human sexuality and (2) clinical experience in the targeted examination of patients.

This holistic approach is the basis of syndyastic sexual therapy, which aims at enhancing the quality of the relationship as a whole and thus increasing the satisfaction of the couple by focussing on the fulfillment of fundamental needs. This releases the potentiality of changing a pathogenic view on sexuality to a salutogenic one and resolving the respective sexual disorder(s). In this process the therapist assists the couple in healing themselves. The same objective also applies to singles, whether temporary or permanent, who can also profit from the syndyastic concept, but need other resources of acceptance and support.

Although it is not claimed to offer a cure-all, it has to be taken into account that medical care is moving incredibly fast in the direction of health maintenance and health enhancement. Here sexual health holds a key position for life quality, which health professionals need to accommodate by helping patients to achieve their desired level of sexual and partnership contentedness.

Berlin, Innsbruck   K. M. Beier, K. K. Loewit

Contents

About the Authors

Klaus M. Beier was born in 1961 in Berlin. He received his MD (1986) and PhD (1988) at the Free University of Berlin and subsequently worked in the Department of Sexology at the University of Kiel, Northern Germany (1988–1996). His main focus in research at that time was forensic sexology, in particular follow-up studies of previously expertly evaluated sexual offenders. Since 1996 he has been working at the Humboldt-University of Berlin as the director of the newly founded Institute of Sexology and Sexual Medicine. This institute is part of the University Hospital Charité, the biggest University Clinic in Europe. This Institute offers lectures and tutorials for undergraduate students of all disciplines such as medicine, psychology, social and cultural sciences, humanities, etc. Professor Beier is in charge of the outpatient clinic of the institute which covers the full range of sexual and gender identity disorders. Since 1997 he has been responsible for the officially accredited post-graduate courses in sexual medicine, training colleagues from other specialized fields such as andrology, endocrinology, general medicine, gynecology, psychiatry, psychosomatics, psychotherapy and urology as well as clinical psychology. His latest research focuses on the prevention of child sexual abuse. The goal is to encourage self-identified undetected pedophiles and hebephiles to seek professional help in order to avoid committing child sexual abuse or engaging with child abusive images on the internet (www.dont-offend.org).

Kurt K. Loewit was born in 1934 in Innsbruck, Austria. He graduated in 1959 from the Medical School of the University of Innsbruck. From 1967 to 1969 he was a Postdoctoral research fellow at the Population Council, Rockefeller University in New York. After his return to Europe, he started lecturing on sexual medicine and introduced the subject into the medical curriculum. Among other study trips, he attended two training seminars at the Masters & Johnson Institute in St. Louis and broadened the therapeutic concept by focusing on the communicative dimension of sexuality. Appointed university professor in 1979, he retired in 1999 from heading the Department of Sexual Medicine at the University Clinic for Medical Psychology and Psychotherapy in Innsbruck. As of 1997 he has cooperated with Prof. K. M. Beier in developing the concept of syndyastic sexual therapy and implementing postgraduate training programs in sexual medicine for physicians and psychologists in Berlin and in Salzburg, Austria.

Chapter 1
A Short Reader for a Holistic Approach on Human Sexuality and Its Disorders

1.1 Sexual Medicine in Clinical Practice: An Overview

Considering the impact of sexuality on the life of every human being and in many ways for society in general, there is no doubt it should get the same attention within the medical and public health care system as other elementary areas of life have long since.

> Wilhelm von Humboldt (1767–1835) wrote already in 1795: It takes but "a small effort of thinking to make the meaning of gender go far further than the restricted sphere it is locked into and allow it to become an immeasurably broad topic."

To achieve this, it is necessary to establish an extensive theory as a basis of an integral therapy, so that sexological ways of thinking and acting can be integrated into clinical practice for the benefit of the patients and can be done in a skilled and competent way.

Definition:

Sexual medicine is involved in prevention, recognition, treatment and reha-
bilitation of disorders and diseases concerning sexual functions, sexual and/or
partnership experiences and behaviour, sexual preferences as well as gender
identity. This also refers to real or threatening sexually delinquent behaviour as
well as traumatization caused by sexual offences. Such disorders and diseases
can be caused by other illnesses and/or their treatment. Partnership aspects
play an important part in diagnosis and therapy.

Specialized knowledge is necessary for diagnosis, classification, prevention, counselling competence and differentiated therapy options concerning disorders of

K. M. Beier, K. K. Loewit, *Sexual Medicine in Clinical Practice*,
DOI 10.1007/978-1-4614-4421-3_1, © Springer Science+Business Media, LLC 2013

sexual function, sexual development, sexual preference, sexual behaviour, sexual re-production as well as gender identity—also if caused by other illnesses and/or their treatment.

An overall view of these different disorders, most of which have been meticulously recorded by internationally valid classification systems (ICD-10 and DSM-IV-TR), are to be found in Chap. 4.

Often, the fact is overlooked that sexuality is not only a personal but also an interpersonal affair, so that there is not always one patient but one *couple* to be dealt with. Keeping in mind that these connections are validated by neurobiological research results, it is of even more relevance that neither somatic medicine nor psychotherapy has theoretically well-founded tools at their disposal with which the *partnership aspects* could adequately be assessed.

Sexual medicine in itself relies on a theoretical concept for diagnostics and ther-apy, which does justice to the neurobiological as well as the psychosocial aspects of sexual relationships. This concept is explained in detail in Chap. 3 and is crucial for the diagnostic assessment of any problem (see Chap. 5). The essential interdis-ciplinary orientation of sexual medicine is dealt with in Chap. 2 and reveals that every one-dimensional approach to sexual disorders—no matter if in a somatic or psychotherapeutic manner—exactly does not fulfil the criteria of sexological practice.

> The bare circumstance that several disciplines in the field of medicine are concerned with sexual disorders does not automatically insure sexological thinking and acting.

In consequence, this also applies to therapy: If the treatment of sexual disorders is carried out without taking the dimension of attachment (see Chap. 3.1) into account and without looking into the situation of the couple concerned, as, for instance, by prescribing a PDE-5-inhibitor for erectile disorder, based only on the information of the male patient involved and not taking into account an own impression gained by talking to the female partner, i.e. the couple as a whole, it could easily lead to no benefit arising for the actual situation of the partnership and thus lead to offending against the medical principle of "nihil nocere".

That is why sexological consultation goes further than a purely functional con-sultation (transmitting functional information and prescribing medication, etc.) by provoking talks about possibly wrong expectations, allowing well-directed sugges-tions concerning behaviour modifications, which necessarily take both partners to work on and achieve results. In chronified disorders, these could be grounds for a sexual therapy (see Chap. 6).

> Just "advice on function" in cases of sexual disorder cannot be considered as sexological counselling!

This does not mean that sexual medicine does not operate with somatic therapy options, whenever there are diagnostic grounds that this may lead to an enhancement of sexual and/or partnership comfort in both partners.

> "Clinical experience demonstrates that sexual dysfunction is rarely a simple performance problem with a simple cure" (see Metz and McCarthy 2007).

Sexual medicine puts priority on the dimension of attachment, derived from scientific findings in evolutionary biology and ethology, showing that mammals, especially primates and certainly humans are "relational" beings programmed with a "social brain", dependent on attachment: their chances of survival depend on the fulfilment of existential elementary needs such as acceptance and belonging. These are most likely to be fulfilled and particularly intensive during body contact in (intimate) relationships providing feelings of comfort and security. All sexological actions are based on'this elementary understanding (see Chaps. 5 and 6).

These basic prerequisites expand all currently known methods of sexological consultation and therapy, mainly based on Masters and Johnson (1966) and are distinguished from these by the explicit reference to fundamental needs of all human beings and the specific assignment or translation of the communicative potential of sexuality.

Thus, the concept of *syndyastic sexual therapy* puts fulfilment of psychosocial fundamental needs into the focus of therapy (see Beier and Loewit 2004), which makes it quite different from all other treatment methods.

This therapeutic concept, which is to be introduced here in detail, aims at two goals: Firstly, to make the patients (best: the couple) aware of the dimension of attachment in sexuality (making them realize that by intimate encounter fundamental needs can be fulfilled) and secondly, to establish a different point of view on sexual arousal. In many cases, this part of sexuality is literally detached from the relationship and is experienced as something impersonal and non-committal. So, while in classical sexual therapy the re-establishment of sexual function was the main priority, in this concept, the stabilization of the partnership is focused on. The re-establishment of sexual function as an expression of "newly gained intimacy" is made easier and at the same time more valuable by new meaning. Therefore, Masters and Johnson's so-called "sensuality training" referred in the first place to the re-establishment of functional impairment, while this new approach employs sensuality training to improve partnership contentedness. This is achieved by feeling acceptance and closeness in terms of the so-called "new experiences" (the couple itself develops and decides on these new experiences mutually), giving them a different meaning than in classical sexual therapy. This calls for new expressions, a new terminology.

Due to the overall significance of fundamental needs in general, this approach tends to easily trigger evident experiences in advice-seeking patients.

One female patient, who was acquainted with both forms of therapy, the classical one and the syndyastic one, put it this way: *I prefer the relationship-centred approach, the other one seems too technical.*

Admittedly, at first sight, this kind of attachment and communication-orientated sexual therapy quite obviously does not seem to reflect the mainstream of today's forms of partnership. However, in cases of disorders it is experienced as coinciding with real longings and hopes, hitting the exact heart of the problems, being helpful and having a healing effect. Often, long "incubation times" precede, before people, i.e. couples finally go seeking help. By being prepared to do this together, for each other, they are demonstrating the crucial meaning of partnership and communication for their chosen life style. The boundaries of therapy are therefore closely linked to the boundaries of the current partnership, finally reached by the boundaries of partnership capabilities themselves. Is the partnership too far damaged or missing altogether (e.g. in serious personality disorders), the syndyastic sexual therapy will find no means of approach and in such cases it might be necessary to take individual psychotherapeutic offers into consideration.

This compendium serves quick orientation covering the clinically most important disorders in sexual medicine concerning their different forms of manifestation and the appropriate diagnostic and therapeutic approach. Based on the general concept of the three dimensions of human sexuality (see Chap. 3.1) special characteristics of each disorder and overlappings are demonstrated—often illustrated by case report examples. Further particularities of each indication area, such as disorders of gender identity (see Chap. 4.3) or disorders of sexual behaviour (see Chap. 4.5) which need to be dealt with in clinical routine, are also concisely characterized and enable medical doctors and psychologists as well as other health care professionals to easily orientate themselves and to initiate adequate actions.

This relates as much to actual knowledge deficits (e.g. concerning disorders of sexual reproduction, see Chap. 4.6), as to new challenges by the internet and the new media, which not only influence "patient knowledge" (e.g. by the enormous opportunities of obtaining information via the internet), but may also influence sexual self-perception, gender-role definition and lastly, sexual preference or sexual behaviour of future generations as well (see p. 7.1). Finally, there are new scientific findings concerning primary prevention of sexual behaviour disorders and sexual traumatization also dealt with in this book (see Chaps. 7.2 and 7.3) in order to widely spread clinically relevant knowledge to the interested public.

Chapter 2
Interdisciplinary References in Sexual Medicine

Sexual medicine by definition includes anthropological, biomedical, psychological and socio-cultural aspects of sexuality and gender. It is by nature interdisciplinary and constantly integrates the know-how from other specialized fields such as general medicine, gynecology, urology, andrology, endocrinology, psychiatry, psychosomatics, psychotherapy as well as from adjoining human sciences, especially biology, psychology, sociology, etc. This corresponds with the large variety of patients: For instance, the diabetes patient complaining of sexual disorders at some stage during his chronic disease (erectile disorder in men, arousal and orgasm problems in women); the hypertonic patient whose medication affects his sexual reactions negatively; the patient suffering from depression, lacking sexual desire (as well as perhaps having to cope with arousal and orgasm difficulties).

All these patients give an impression of the mentioned diversity as does the young man with sexual performance anxiety; the couple, whose unresolved conflicts or struggles for power within their partnership lead to sexual symptoms; the woman, who suffers pain during intercourse caused by lack of lubrication after menopause, etc. (Fig. 2.1).

In addition to that there is the enormous and growing significance of disorders of sexual preference (paraphilias, see Chap. 4.4) and disorders of sexual behaviour (dissexuality, see Chap. 4.5), having currently become an issue of attention in the media due to the revealed cases of sexual abuse at institutions (such as the church), which are now able to be precisely diagnosed, provided that the necessary expertise in sexual medicine is deployed.

Looking at the available specialized preventive and therapeutic measures which are able to indeed prevent sexual offences, makes the connection to the criminal justice system evident. This is true anyway for expert opinion activity concerning legally registered sexual delinquents.

It is a matter of great concern for sexual medicine to provide other disciplines with its specialized knowledge, making a contribution to help improve public sexual health. This is most effective if further development of sexual disorders can be hindered or the occurrence of sexual traumatization can be prevented.

When the increasing numbers of disorders in sexual reproduction (see Chap. 4.6) are considered, including the often massive effects of involuntary childlessness on

K. M. Beier, K. K. Loewit, *Sexual Medicine in Clinical Practice,*
DOI 10.1007/978-1-4614-4421-3_2, © Springer Science+Business Media, LLC 2013

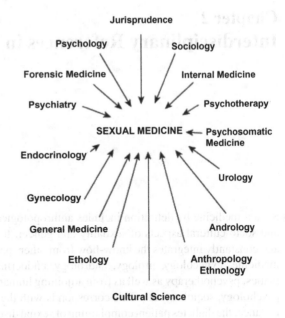

Fig. 2.1 Interdisciplinary references in sexual medicine (p. 7)

sexual and partnership comfort (see Beier et al. 2005), the spectrum of sexual disorders is broadened and the challenges to sexual medicine become apparent.

However, the contributions of various adjoining disciplines to the significance of sexual medicine confirm anthropological findings that human beings are relational beings programmed with a "social brain", relying on loving care and acceptance. All this is general knowledge. It is not only that many patients/couples do not see the connection between attachment, partnership-comfort and psychosocial basic needs on the one hand and sexuality on the other, even a great number of professional counsellors within the health system do not estimate this adequately either (see Chap. 3).

The inevitable interdisciplinarity of sexual medicine is automatically given by the fact that sexuality is an interpersonal event. On the one hand, this leads to the necessity of relying on basic knowledge concerning communication, partnership and social relationship issues, etc. On the other hand, just as much, consequently integrating the partner into the assessment procedure as well as into the therapy itself.

Only by heeding this "pair aspect" and carrying out the work with both partners consequently from the beginning, the prevailing mutual influences and interferences within a partnership are taken into account, otherwise, the reality of the couple in their partnership is missed. These "pair dynamics" can have a positive boosting effect and a salutogenic impact or they can activate and maintain a negative "downwards spiral" and a self-reinforcing pathogenic vicious circle. Figure 2.2 using the example of an erectile disorder, illustrates how this interaction of overlapping vicious circles in the couple itself can lead to disadvantages for both partners and their relationship on the functional as well as on the partnership level.

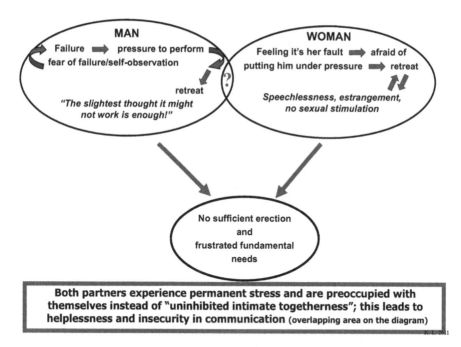

Fig. 2.2 Overlapping vicious circles in erectile dysfunction (p.8)

An interruption of interaction perpetuating existing disorders can only be achieved by specialized diagnostic assessment, meaning that specialized knowledge and skills are called for, which are in no way mediated during current medical or psychological training, as these concentrate on diagnostic assessment of individual—and exactly not interpersonal—disorder conditions. The same applies to therapy, which consequently would need to begin with the couple from the start. Neither in postgraduate training for physicians nor in psychotherapeutic supplementary courses are there any systematic approaches underlining the necessity of specialized qualifying measures for sexual medicine and the syndyastic sexual therapy (see Chap. 6.7).

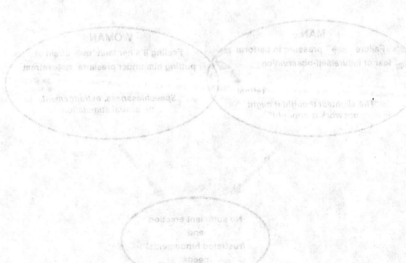

Chapter 3
Basic Understanding of Human Sexuality

Sexuality can be defined as a biologically, psychologically and socially determined quality of experience in human beings, which is formed by the unique development of a person's own life history.

Generally speaking, sexuality refers to everything concerning being female and being male, sexual identity and gender roles, obviously sexual organs (i.e. the gonads) and their functions, bearing in mind that apart from the genital part of sexual experience and behaviour, a crucial role is allocated to all five senses and the brain as the control centre. For didactic reasons, it should be differentiated between the biological, psychological and social aspects, but in reality these are not separateable, meaning they are non-existent on their own. By now, even patients distinguish between biological-organic or psychological causes of their disorders—the first mentioned being real and acceptable, whereas the second seem to bear the odium of being mentally ill in a psychiatric way, thus causing resistance and opposition.

That is why, in certain cases, patients have to be convinced about the existence of a biopsychosocial unity and entirety of the human being in its sexuality, before integral treatment is possible.

3.1 The Three Dimensions of Sexuality

From a practical point of view, one can speak of the multi-functionalism of sexuality comprising single aspects interacting with one another which are distinguished from one another by following terms:

- The *dimension of desire* encompasses sexuality in all conceivable ways of experiencing and increasing desire by sexual stimulation.
- The *dimension of reproduction* stands for the significance of sexuality in reproduction.
- The *dimension of attachment* emphasizes the importance of sexuality for the fulfilment of biopsychosocial fundamental needs for acceptance, closeness, warmth and security by sexual communication in partnership (see Beier and Loewit 2004; Beier et al. 2005).

K. M. Beier, K. K. Loewit, *Sexual Medicine in Clinical Practice*,
DOI 10.1007/978-1-4614-4421-3_3, © Springer Science+Business Media, LLC 2013

In fantasy, as well as in reality, these three dimensions of sexuality are experienced and valued differently according to different life stages.

The *dimension of reproduction* with the beginning of puberty (onset of menstruation, first-ever ejaculation) can waver between being overrated on one hand and completely lacking significance on the other, taking the gender difference into account, that males are principally capable of reproduction even at an older age, while the reproductive capability in women diminishes at the stage of menopause.

The *dimension of attachment*, the socially communicative dimension, experiences its individual character at the earliest life stage, as an infant, in the sense of a non-genital-centered pre-form of infant sexuality and reaches a high quality very early in life, influencing further life, but more often than not remaining unreflected.

The *dimension of desire* begins with arising physical sensations of desire/lust, probably already intrauterine, definitely in very early infancy (the so-called infant masturbation) and generally keeps up its significance beginning at sexual maturity for the rest of the life-span.

Of the three dimensions, the *reproductive dimension* of sexuality is the phylogenetically oldest in higher animals. At the stage of the single-celled organism, the so-called parasexual processes such as conjugation, a kind of mating, exchanging of genetic material between two cells, does not serve reproduction, rather a genetic recombination, providing raw material for evolution. Multiplication occurs asexually. Only the more sophisticated multi-cellular organisms combined genetic recombination (during germ cell maturation) and multiplication to operate reproduction as we know it.

For women, this dimension is limited to the time span of reproductive capability extending from puberty to menopause; it is also dependant on biographical decisions, making it optional. The availability of reliable contraceptive methods on one hand, and the progress of reproductive medicine on the other, has made it possible to separate the dimension of reproduction from the other two dimensions of desire and attachment.

The *dimension of desire* provides sexuality with the unique sensual experience of sexual arousal and orgasm, which distinguishes it from other human experience. It establishes the motivational quality of sexuality and simultaneously provides the impulse and reward of sexual behaviour. The dimension of desire can predominate in subjective experience in autoeroticism and in experienced erotic interactions, passion and ecstasy.

In our dualistically organized Western countries, historically hostile in their attitude towards body and sensuality, this dimension has always been an area of tension between condemnation and glorification. It can be an isolated experience, without any connection to the reproductive dimension and the attachment dimension of sexuality. It is, however, difficult to view this dimension completely on its own, because it is so closely connected to the other dimensions and is obviously influenced by various factors outside and within the realm of sexuality. Current media, pornography and sex industries propagate a one-sided predomination of the desire dimension, forcing the other dimensions of sexuality into the background. At the same time, it is a fact that currently, the most widespread sexual disorder happens to be *lack* of sexual desire.

The *dimension of attachment* is established later in evolutionary development, only after the stage of reptiles, in birds and mammals, particularly primates. These social or bonding functions of sexuality, of which many people are not aware, are indeed no human invention.

In the animal kingdom, sexuality has been attributed to social significance, to enhancing pair and group bonding in the sense of a change in meaning and function (see Wickler 1969, 1971, Wickler and Seibt 1984). In human beings—distinguishing themselves from their primate relatives mainly by the capability of speech and creating culture—the attachment dimension of sexuality specifically becomes one with a communication function: Attachment develops by communication, so communication and attachment are interchangeable terms. With reference to the fact that "you cannot not communicate" (Watzlawick et al. 1969) "you cannot not interact" in relationships, and therefore, the function of social attachment in sexuality is an obligatory and life-long relevant function. At the same time, this social function illustrates the specific human elements of sexuality.

Thus, for mankind today, the dimension of attachment is without doubt an integral and essential element of sexuality. Its huge significance derives from the fact that humans are relational beings programmed with a "social brain".

In their attempt to conceptualize this by definition, Beier and Loewit (2004) use the term *syndyastic* dimension of sexuality (i.e. a more specific term referring to the attachment dimension, transferred from the Greek term *syndyasticós* employed by Aristotle to describe the human disposition of living in pairs) thus expressing the significance of fulfilment of fundamental biopsychosocial needs of acceptance, closeness, security and protection by sexual communication within partnership. Next to the dimensions of desire and reproduction, this dimension needs to be explored into separately, in order to trace *syndyastic deprivation* in the patient/couple or to find out about the *syndyastic functional level* of the partnership.

3.2 Neurobiological Findings

Neurobiological findings also show clearly, in which great proportion the brain is a system particularly adapted to and dependent on attachment and how attachment can actually influence genes:

> Various neurobiologically installed systems, e.g. the mirror neurons or the activation of the attachment hormone oxytocin show, that not only our emotional feelings, but also the neurobiology of the brain is a system, adapted to and dependent on interpersonal relationships (see Bauer 2005).

Today, neuro-imaging methods are able to show (see Bartels and Zeki 2004) that the same brain regions are deactivated, for instance regions participating in socially critical judgments in the prefrontal cortex when mothers are shown pictures of their children as well as seeing pictures of their spouses (compared with pictures of known, but not beloved persons as control subjects). Seemingly, the functions for anxiety and rejection, functionally-anatomically located in the amygdala, are deactivated at the same time. This means that any apprehension concerning the partner is "turned off" in order to enable close interaction (presumably the origin of the traditional proverb "love is blind"). At the same time, parts of the rewarding system are activated and release the so-called endorphins. By this, not only trust is enhanced and making contact made easier, but also feelings of happiness are stimulated and distress is markedly reduced on the whole. This would explain the assumption of earlier authors who did not have neuro-imaging methods as evidence, such as the observations of Balint (1965) about the "primeval forms of love" as being the core and basis of adult intimacy, or why A. Montagu (1987) called sexual interaction between adults "in some ways a recapitulation of the tender love between mother and child".

At the same time, data from neuro-sciences suggest that in triggering directly physiologically observable sexual reactions, besides higher parts such as the limbic system, basal cerebral areas close to the anatomical midline (next to mid-brain structures) play a decisive role in causing these processes. Here, the area preoptica of the hypothalamus seems to be of central importance and in animal experiments increased activity in this core region, anatomically connected with other hypothalamic regions, has been observed during sexual activity. Steroid hormones modulate the activity of the area preoptica; experiments on both male and female animal behaviour showed selective activation in sexually promising or coitus-relevant situations (see Pfaff 1999). In human beings, this core is "wired" so that nasally uptaken androgen or oestrogen metabolites can be recognized as important signals. Activation is dependent on sexual orientation and not on gender: androgen metabolites activate core regions in women who are oriented towards men, and in male-oriented men, while in men who are female-orientated this region is activated by oestrogen metabolites (see Savic et al. 2005). The dependence of central sexual activation patterns on sexual orientation (and not on gender) was shown by Ponseti et al. (2006) for visual stimuli.

3.3 The Communicative Function of Sexuality

From the very beginning of life, man's fundamental needs for acceptance, security, trust, warmth and closeness can only be satisfied in relationships (Bowlby 1969–1980; Brisch 1999). During infancy this is accomplished by body contact and the emotional experience of being taken care of, for instance by the sheltering manner in which an infant is held during breastfeeding. By this parental loving care the modus of satisfying psychosocial fundamental needs by skin contact is learned by the infant and reinforced on a *neuronal level*, the way all processes of learning elementary skills generally are (see Rüegg 2003).

Hüther (2005, p. 91 ff.) describes the neurobiological foundations for de-anxiety and stress management by empathic relationships:

> So we repeatedly experienced how anxiety disappeared, when someone was close to us, who gave us security and shelter with their warmth, someone who loved us (...). These tracks were treaded again and again and the feeling, that we are safe with a beloved person was engraved deeply into the brain of every human being.

Feelings transmitted by interaction and body language determine human development from birth onward and remain a core characteristic of partnership organization: At first, they are not dependent on genital involvement, but indeed allow deep satisfaction obtained by skin and eye contact as well as by all other senses. They are therefore the first dimension of "sexual" experience, broadened later in life by the option of genital-sexual communication.

Along with sexual maturity, sexuality now becomes the most intensive form of body language in a genital way. Basically, similar to every behaviour, sexual behaviour also sends signals engaging all senses, facial expression, gestures, body composure, etc. which can at first be ambiguous and liable to be misunderstood. Whether an embrace means use of violence, physical detention, captivation, or whether it means passionate caring, closeness, deeply experienced contact or being held onto, etc. is dependent on the quality of the relationship. So, for instance in a loving partnership and irrespective in principle of sexual orientation the physical behaviour during "sex" can be experienced as intimate attention, being respected and desired, being the centre of perception and affection, being close to someone, being accepted and held, being open for one another, mutual indulgence, feeling one's own body with all-over intensity and other "translations" of experience, such as they are verbalized by couples, who in therapy have discovered the dimension of sensuality in sexual communication for themselves. For instance: "Now I can transmit our closeness of soul onto the physical level". What used to be just "sex" has now obtained a personal significance: "Now it is more like "we" are sleeping together, it used to be just an ordinary sexual act".

In everyday practice, most patients do not perceive sexuality as part of their communication process. They understand "sex" and "love" as two different fields of life and experience, not really having much to do with one another. Table 3.1 gives an overview on typical statements made by patients who express this attitude compared with opinions of patients after treatment.

This integrated understanding of sexuality can give access to and become basis for a mutual view of the world of sexuality in any particular partnership. The term "sleeping together" now expresses what used to be only associated with love and tenderness, but not necessarily with "sex", and was therefore often missed.

Indeed, even authors who place "sexual functioning in the context of love as an attachment bond" and thus come very close to the concept of syndyastics, still follow definitions of adult attachment theory dividing love into three separate behavioural systems: attachment, caregiving and sexuality. Even though the attachment system "is considered to be preeminent and provides the scaffolding for the development and enactment of the other two", sexuality remains a separate, yet connected,

Table 3.1 Patients' quotations on isolated and integrated sexuality

Isolated sexuality (not perceived on a communicational level)	Integrated sexuality (consciously applied as a way of communication)
I could do without sex without missing anything	On this level, sex is a way of reaching me
Always the same procedure: direct foreplay … sleeping away afterwards	It's deeper than just sex—not only him reducing his arousal. I respond differently to his ejaculation—it was something like pleasure
Sex was physical sports—nothing more	Now it's more like *us* sleeping together
Sex does nothing for me. When sex begins, I retreat	For the first time my thoughts were involved—I didn't think about anything else, that was liberating
Sex was a one-way street to orgasm	You were different, you connected more to me
I could live without sex, but not without love, tenderness and warmth	Romance is revived, it is like being married for not more that 6 months
Sex drive—I don't know what that is. I need you to be there, hugging me and caressing me, without *it* being there	Now, for the first time I have experienced sexual intercourse and cuddling not as two different things
There are more important aspects to a partnership than sex	I have never looked at it that way—I was not aware of it, but it had been inside of me all the time
Sex just belongs to a partnership	For us that is a completely revolutionary insight

system (Johnson and Zuccarini 2010). In the syndyastic sexual therapy, sexuality is considered as the sexual form of expressing and enacting attachment, i.e. "proximity-seeking, safety, emotional connection", etc. and thus is integrated as 'sexually embodied love', not something separate, albeit facilitated by love. The above statements elucidate and corroborate this deciding and salutogenic distinction, once it has been completely understood.

> By overcoming the deep rift between affection and love on one side and sex(uality) on the other, current "normal sexual conduct" or even a pathogenic, psycho-toxic interpretation of sexuality, can once more or for the first time turn into a salutogenic, meaning-full perception, quite a source of lust and happiness in life.

This is true—quite regardless of sexual orientation—not only for sexual communication in couples, but also for communication in the widest sense of the word by "sexual body language" (not necessarily meaning sexual communication involving genitals) in single persons—single by choice or involuntarily—or persons who have become single again by separation. And it is also true for "love towards oneself", the autoerotic communication in the relationship to oneself.

The general aim of this therapy, principally understood as a partnership-therapy, is the development and/or the restoration of the salutogenic effect of sexuality, i.e. it is not restricted to the isolated restoration of disturbed sexual function(s), but strives to improve partnership contentment on the whole. The regaining of adequate erection capability, for instance does not automatically restore frustrated fundamental needs within the partnership.

This way, the focus of attention is relocated from the dysfunctions towards the partnership and its issues, and consequently towards the partner, who gains the feeling of being perceived and being a person in the centre of interest: The coitus can, for instance reach a point of "mutual achievement", different from the attitude of one person being absorbed in his/her own sexual function (will my erection be sufficient? Or will I reach orgasm?).

Exactly by this attitude, sexual functioning is relieved from performance pressure and failure anxiety is significantly relaxed, making their compensation easier. This objective is in coherence with findings by Kleinplatz and Menard (2007), referred to as *building blocks towards optimal sexuality*:

According to an interview-study of men and women involved in long-term partnerships, the relevant "building blocks" of optimal sexuality are as follows:

1. Being present (intensely focused attention)
2. Authenticity
3. Intense emotional connection
4. Sexual and erotic intimacy (giving themselves and each other permission "to indulge as well as to be indulgent"
5. Communication
6. Transcendence ("It leaves you bigger than you were before").

This approach is principally relevant for other indications of sexual therapy as well, for instance gender identity disorders and paraphilias.

Such an approach, however, applies also to other medical disciplines beyond sexual medicine and should generally be more regarded in considerations concerning pathogenesis and treatment of diseases in general. This concerns the pathogenic consequences of syndyastic deprivation, but most of all the resources lying in effective satisfaction of fundamental needs. Its salutogenic potential should be principally stimulated and supported by all medical specialties. Then there is an opportunity that the meaning of relationship as being a place of experiencing uninhibited acceptance and the deactivation of anxiety that goes with it, security and distress decrease (along with the definition of sexuality as being an intensive transmitter of this kind of experience) is given a key position within the therapy itself. This is what happens in sexual medicine and its therapeutic principle—the syndyastic sexual therapy.

In sexual therapy, whenever a new and salutogenic understanding is aimed at, the doctor or therapist as an individual plays a crucial role, because his/her personal attitude will make an impression on the patient(s). This matter of personality would not be of such importance if it were only about conveying techniques or prescribing medication for regaining sexual functions and if it were not about questions concerning a new sense of understanding.

In the course of this approach, it cannot be a question of technique *or* relationship, physical desire *or* satisfaction of fundamental needs; it concerns the general holistic approach. Particularly in relationships and communication, 'techniques' can be of great advantage and very helpful. In true, authentic communication 'sexual desire' can be liberated from cultural taboos and can develop in an un-inhibited way, because there is no reason to be in any way ashamed of true (shame-free) communication.

> No technique, no arousal-raising trick, and no medication will be able to compensate the missing meaning and authentic communication needed with self and other, where function disorders are connected with being offended and lacking communication within the partnership.

As a result, only those health professionals who approve of the concept of the syndyastic sexual therapy and are convinced of the possibility of salutogenic sexual communication are in a position to offer authentic ideas to a couple in need. Whether or not they accept these offers relies entirely on the couple itself. Among the various methods of treatment for sexual disorders, the connection between fulfilment of psychosocial fundamental needs as a given basis for partnership quality and sexuality itself as an extremely strong expression of communicating this fulfilment is only consequently achieved in the concept of syndyastic sexual therapy. It aims at and achieves this fulfilment, and therefore, it needs to be basically approved of by the therapist.

This clearly underlines the particular necessity for self-reflection in the therapist, also of self-awareness and supervision concerning questions of sexuality and partnership, because these issues concern everyone personally. This applies especially in situations when the counselling or therapy situation becomes eroticized or sexualized, i.e. more in one-to-one therapy than in couple-therapy. The problem here would lie in the fact of overstepping the boundaries and in the abuse of the patient, not in the fact of erotic feelings or feelings of attraction as such. Sexual interaction between client and therapist is always professional malpractice.

However, sexuality can generally not only be seen in a positive, but also in a negative destructive sense, as a means of punishment, of power abuse (in the sense of subjugation, rape and abuse) or even as a weapon in war, and as "antithesis" as reversal of experiencing tenderness and love it may embody the destructive relationship, which always has to be taken into account in sexual disorders. Similarly, promiscuitive behaviour or sexual episodes lacking relationship (e.g. one-night stands, prostitution, surrogate partner)—driven on by rushes of sexual arousal and lust—may also feign feelings of experiencing acceptance, contact, closeness and security, but only on the physical level or on the level of genital-orgastic drive.

Fulfilment of fundamental needs is, so to speak, "technically feigned", and therefore frustrated. In certain circles of youth subculture, quick "unconnected" sex can reach the status of a surrogate drug to compensate unfulfilled fundamental needs.

Therefore, stimulating the desire-system, while at the same time frustrating the fulfilment of fundamental needs in a relationship could be termed "syndyastic deprivation" (see Beier and Loewit 2004). This is definitely a new challenge for sexual medicine—but at the same time also for society in general (see Chap. 7.)

Chapter 4
The Spectrum of Sexual Disorders

The suggested categories of the clinical classification systems ICD-10 (WHO 1993) and DSM-IV-TR (APA 2000) are purely descriptive concepts which fail to do justice to the complexity of human sexuality.

Already, by taking into account the sexologically required differentiation of the three dimensions of sexuality, the inadequacy of such categorization is unmasked. Thus, sexual disorders cannot only influence the dimension of desire, but very likely the dimension of attachment as well and hence not only the disturbed sexual function but moreover the disturbance of partnership comfort turns out to be the actual reason for suffering.

> According to present knowledge, chronic lack of feelings of security transmitted by body communication (frustration of psychosocial fundamental needs) increases the probability of developing psychological and physical disorders. Furthermore, it hinders overcoming prevailing illnesses (Egle et al. 1997).

The symptoms presented by patients seen in clinical practice are usually described as "psychosomatic disorders", "depressive state of mood", "anxiety and/or nervous restlessness", i.e., "nervous anxiety, tension and restlessness" or additionally as "emotionally caused state of restlessness". Therefore, it can be assumed that in many areas of medicine male and female patients with varying disorders or dysfunctions consult a practitioner, because—again for different reasons—of a lack of availability of a functioning and therefore emotionally stabilizing intimate attachment. Also, included are chronically ill or older persons, suffering from psychosocial destabilization due to reduced opportunities for social contacts.

This explains why very different symptoms can dominate the clinical impression and, as a result, various medical disciplines may come into contact with the patients concerned: Orthopedics for muscle tension; gynecology and urology for pelvic floor tensions, disturbances of micturition, etc.; general practice for symptoms of the autonomic nervous system; psychiatry for intrapsychic tension or states of depression; or andrology concerning involuntary childlessness. Also, sexual dysfunction may perhaps be only one of the many possible symptoms (apart from, of course, sexual

K. M. Beier, K. K. Loewit, *Sexual Medicine in Clinical Practice,*
DOI 10.1007/978-1-4614-4421-3_4, © Springer Science+Business Media, LLC 2013

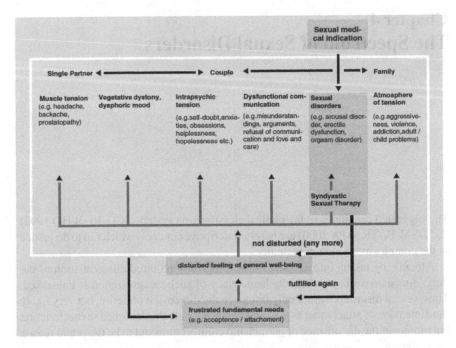

Fig. 4.1 Connection between psychological fundamental needs and various symptoms

disorders caused by illness, e.g., condition after paraplegia). The special quality of sexological therapy options (see Chap. 6) lies in the fact that it deals explicitly with the actual roots (the frustrated fundamental needs) of possible causes at a level not reached elsewhere, while it aims at restoring the feeling of complete attachment by physical acceptance through intimacy with the partner, which also has curative effects on symptoms and positive consequences in other areas of life (Fig. 4.1).

Therefore, even in the case of spinal pains, (e.g., as a symptom of muscle tension, possibly caused by distress in an unsatisfactory partnership) having been successfully cured by an orthopedist, there is nevertheless no change on the level of fundamental needs and partnership comfort. Potential frustration of these needs is neither revealed nor resolved and may lead to a recurrence of the former symptoms or cause other impairments.

Notwithstanding these limited and only partially useful systematic categorizations, clinically significant sexual disorders are compactly characterized as follows, along with their coding definitions—according to the international classification systems (ICD-10 and DSM-IV-TR; see Ahlers et al. 2005):

1. Disorders of sexual function (ICD-10: F 52.0 ff.; DSM-IV-TR: 302.71 ff.).
2. Disorders of sexual development (ICD-10:F 66.0 ff.; coded in the generalized category "not otherwise specified" in DSM-IV-TR: 302.9).

   (a) Disorder of sexual maturity.
   (b) Disorder of sexual orientation.

    (c) Disorder of sexual identity.
    (d) Disorder of sexual relationship.

3. Disorders of gender identity (ICD-10: F 64.0; DSM-IV-TR: 302.85).
4. Disorders of sexual preference/paraphilias (ICD-10: F 65.O ff.; DSM IV-TR: 302.81 ff.).
5. Disorders of sexual behavior/dissexuality (coded in the generalized category "not otherwise specified" in ICD-10: F 63.8 and DSM-IV-TR: 312.30).
6. Disorders of sexual reproduction (coded in the generalized category "not otherwise specified" in ICD-10: F 69.0 and DSM-IV-TR: 309.9).

It must be kept in mind that each sexual disorder is itself capable of causing other disorders which are encoded (e.g., chronic prostatitis, fluor genitalis, etc.), but they can also occur overlapping with one another: Disorders of sexual function are very often closely linked to disorders of sexual relationship. For those disorders of sexual preference which are not integrated into self-concept this is regularly the case (see Chap. 4.4), and there, just as regularly, also disorders of sexual function (e.g., erectile disorder) arise. This, again, underlines the serious impact of unfulfilled psychosocial fundamental needs, which play, in the end, a key role in all sexologically relevant disorders.

4.1 Disorders of Sexual Functions

The sexual response cycle can be subdivided into the following phases: desire, excitement, orgasm, and resolution and each one of these phases can be disturbed (Masters and Johnson 1966).

According to Masters and Johnson (1966), this subdivision applies to both sexes, although there are time differences to be noted. The whole course of reaction is more rapid in males, which may lead to problems for the female in reaching orgasm. The (statistic) curves of male sexual reaction are more stereotype, whilst those of females show larger variability. During increasing age, in males only, a longer lasting refractory period is recorded, while females are readily able to experience multiple orgasms, which make them, so to speak, the "stronger sex" as far as sexual potency is concerned. A different model for female sexual reaction was introduced by Basson (2000, 2002). For males its validity would have to be proven, at least for some of them. She is under the impression—supplemental to Masters and Johnsons' concept and particularly where long-term partnerships are concerned—that the sexual reaction of a woman, i.e., the awakening of her libido, is more based on her needs for intimacy and partnership comfort than her needs for physical sexual excitement and satisfaction. The traditional concept of sexual reaction ignores (for women) essential components of sexual comfort such as: trust, intimacy, respect, communication,

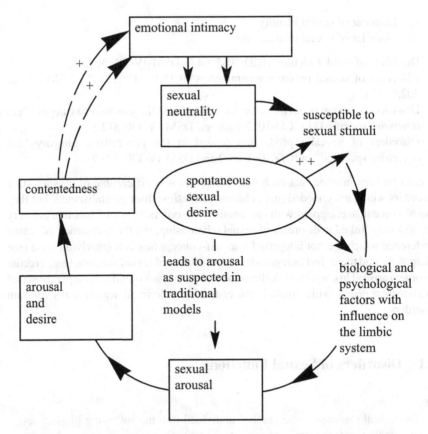

Fig. 4.2 Sexual reaction cycle. (Basson 2002)

affection, and happiness based on sensual tenderness. This causes sexual libido to be understood more as a response to primarily nonsexual needs and not so much as a spontaneous or primary incident (which, particularly in young women it can be, too). Starting from a state of "sexual neutrality" but in need for experiencing intimacy, an "awareness of a nonsexual need to be sexual" arises which then consciously turns into a deliberate choice to experience sexual stimulation. This, in turn, intensifies the experience of intimacy, increases sexual arousal, and ultimately leads to physical well-being, with or without orgasm. This approach underlines the high value of fundamental needs, but does not look at genital sexuality as a means of body language-communication which fulfills exactly these needs at the same time (Fig. 4.2).

The prevalence rates of sexual dysfunctions are high and held responsible for "high degrees of stress and inter-personal difficulties" (DSM-IV-TR) and their impact on health and well-being (WHO) is of great practical relevance.

In a representative random sample of 18–59-year-old US-Americans, Laumann et al. (1999) found that 5 % of the test persons had low sexual desire disorder, 5 %

Table 4.1 Disorders of sexual function according to ICD-10/DSM-IV-TR

	ICD-10		DSM-IV-TR
F52.0	Lack or loss of sexual desire	302.71	Hypoactive sexual desire disorder
F52.1	Sexual aversion and lack of sexual enjoyment	302.79	Sexual aversion disorder
F52.2	Failure of genital response	302.72	Female sexual arousal disorder
F52.3	Orgasmic dysfunction	302.73	Female orgasmic disorder
F52.4	Premature ejaculation	302.75	Premature ejaculation
F52.5	Nonorganic vaginismus	306.51	Vaginismus
F52.6	Nonorganic dyspareunia	302.76	Dyspareunia
F52.7	Excessive sexual drive	–	
F52.8	Other sexual dysfunction, not caused by other disorder or disease	–	
F52.9	Unspecified sexual dysfunction, not caused by other disorder or disease	302.70	Sexual disorder NOS

erectile disorder and 21 % orgasmic disorder in the form of premature ejaculation. In international comparison, results were partly concurrent, but partly showed significant intercultural variations, which is attributed to the biopsychosocial roots of such disorders (Laumann et al. 2005). Since then, several studies have also verified the negative impact of sexual disorders on partnership and quality of life (Chevret et al. 2004; Rosen et al. 2004; Fisher et al. 2005; Abraham et al. 2008).

In accordance, epidemiologically, in males, premature ejaculation is dominant as well as erectile disorder and failure anxiety. In addition, in the last 20–30 years there has been a substantial increase in hypoactive sexual desire disorder. Anorgasmia and dyspareunia very rarely occur, as is true for real disorders of ejaculation such as retarded, retrograde, and deficient ejaculation (for an overview see Table 4.1). In these, the clinical assessment is crucial concerning fertility: In the case of retrograde ejaculation (caused by malfunction of the innervation of the neck of the bladder), the sperm can be retrieved from the bladder; in failing ejaculation, invasive methods of reproductive medicine need to be applied.

In reported female sexual disorders, low sexual desire is top of the list, showing a drastic increase in the last 2–3 decades followed by anorgasmia, lubrication disturbances, and dyspareunia, although the arousal and orgasm disturbances have distinctly receded during the same time period (see Schmidt 1996). Primarily somatic causes such as cardiovascular or metabolic diseases, nerve lesions, influence of medication, etc. do not seem to affect the sexual functions in females as much as in males.

Similar to psychological and behavioral disorders, all sexual disorders reveal biological and psychological, as well as social conditions, so that only a holistic viewpoint on these factors guarantees an appropriate description and consequently effective treatment. As sexual difficulties do not only affect the patient, but also have an impact on the well-being of the partner involved, treatment should principally be carried out with both partners. Moreover, all dysfunctions can occur independently from other illnesses and disorders, or they may result from other illnesses and/or their treatment.

Disorders of sexual function—according to DSM-IV-TR (APA 2000)—can be distinguished as follows:

Lifelong type (present since the onset of sexual functioning),
Acquired type (develops after a period of normal functioning),
Generalized type (not limited to certain types of stimulation, situations or partners), and
Situational type (limited to certain types of stimulation, situations or partners).

Ultimately, disorders of sexual function can be divided into two groups: The already-mentioned "direct" (meaning obvious straightforward) ones and the so-called "indirect" ones. These cover unspecific psychosomatic or somatization symptoms, which can be caused by various conditions, among them possibly some connected with sexuality, which can only be uncovered by careful clinical assessment and holistic diagnostics involving both partners. This has immense clinical relevance: in gynecology, for instance, pelvic pain or parametropathy, the so-called "psychogenic" bleedings, problems of micturition, vulvar itching, fluor genitalis, etc. can become unsolvable problems for the patient and the physician; and in urology there are such issues as chronic prostatitis or prostatopathy causing undefined pain in the anogenital region.

Practically, every clinical medical department is in charge of patients possibly suffering from a sexual disorder through an illness and/or its treatment. Primarily cardiovascular diseases, (heart failure, coronary heart disease, myocardial infarction, and hypertonia) are the main ones which are sexologically relevant. In addition, there are metabolic diseases such as diabetes mellitus, serious general illnesses, especially cancer, locomotor restrictions (e.g., arthritis), neurological illnesses such as multiple sclerosis or morbus Parkinson, but also neurologically related handicaps, psychiatric illnesses such as anxiety disorder or depression, and also mental retardation and finally gynecological and urogenital illnesses.

An independent specific coding of illness-related or treatment-related sexual disorders is as complicated in DSM-IV-TR as it is in ICD-10. In ICD-10, the primary illness is coded separately, while in DSM-IV-TR the disorder is identified, but the primary illness has to be filled in by free text. The multitudes of possible reasons for the development of erectile disorders caused by illness or treatment are shown in Fig. 4.3.

4.1.1 Disorders of Sexual Desire

Disorders of sexual desire can appear as lack of interest or as loss of desire (hypoactive sexual desire disorder; ICD-10: F 52.0; DSM-IV-TR: 302.71), in the worst case (definitely more often in women) as sexual aversion (ICD-10: F 52.10; DSM IV-TR: 302.79) up to sexual phobia accompanied by vegetative signs of repulsion and disgust as well as fury, tremor, nausea, tachycardia, etc.

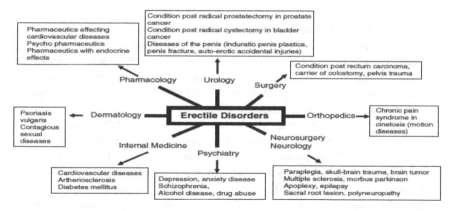

Fig. 4.3 Erectile disorders caused by illnesses and/or their treatment

They are not genital function disorders in a strict sense, but definitely do influence the genital functions—also those of the partner—as well.

Hypoactive sexual desire disorders are becoming an ever-growing problem in men seeking sexological treatment, although the patients themselves often state erectile disorder as their main reason for seeking help. The cause is often found to be hidden, frequently revealing subdepressive conditions of exhaustion (with and without substance abuse), disharmonies in partnership and—always recurrent—disorders of sexual preference. Organic causes (testosterone deficit, hyperprolactinemia, side effects of medication) are definitely significant for differential diagnosis, but are sometimes overestimated in somatomedical literature.

Finally, there will be need to discuss the influence of chemicals with hormonal effects from the environment (e.g., estrogens, i.e., xeno-estrogens, meaning natural and industrial substances with estrogen-like effects), having been detected influencing reproduction in animals and humans (see Schlenker 2004; Fraser 2006; Wagner and Öhlmann 2009).

Case Report 1 The 37-year-old patient was referred by a urologist after not having found any somatic causes for an hypoactive sexual desire disorder. The patient complained of a similar course in all past relationships and was "quite sure", that the present partner was actually "the right one". All the more reason for him to be worried that, after the usual "beginning euphoria", even here the rate of sexual contacts was receding rapidly. His girlfriend did not want the partnership to become permanent, if this problem was not solved. He wanted to move in with her and establish a family. The 3 years younger girlfriend reported having experienced obvious desire in all previous partnerships and was very worried about the complete "lack of enthusiasm" in this one. Because of this, she sees no basis for a long-term partnership, although she is very fond of her present boyfriend and gets along with him "very well" in all other fields of life. This patient was diagnosed with hypoactive sexual desire disorder, as well as erectile disorder, each of the situational type (normal function during masturbation—one to three times per week).

The assessment of the sexual preference structure revealed a foot fetishistic pattern, not integrated into his own self-concept. He had known, since adolescence, that a slender woman's foot had always been the relevant stimulus in the fantasies accompanying masturbation, but he rejected these for himself and was sure to be able to split them off, when being in sexual contact with "the right woman". So, during sexual interaction with his girlfriend, he was intensely focused on not fantasizing the ideal woman's foot (which, by the way, his girlfriend does not have) and this made him tense and "stressed out". Here is a disorder of sexual preference which led to sexual function disorder and resulted in a disorder of sexual relationship (for treatment see Chap. 6.2).

In women, stress can be created by failure of not fulfilling the alleged "normal" picture, meaning that of the sexually interested and sexually active woman, also a feeling of guilt toward the partner ("I know it's all my fault!"), which again has a negative effect on self-esteem, even if it is not visible on the surface.

Sexual intercourse is still an option, even in cases of lack of sexual desire. Depending on the general situation, it can be taken for love, just tolerated, borne, or repelled ("Hurry up and get it over and done with") or it can increase the sexual aversion so far as to make the act unbearable. In any case, it has massive influence on partnership dynamics and quality, both partners are frustrated as far as the fulfillment of their fundamental needs is concerned and sexuality loses its salutogenic potential.

Case Report 2 The 35-year-old (female) bank clerk had "taken off her wedding ring" during the last holiday with the family, because she felt her partnership had reached a low-point. During these holidays, her 2 years older husband (insurance agent) had not given any attention at all to her or their son; he had just followed "his own interests". At the same time, he always complained that they hardly had any sexual contact any more, even though she "felt" like it happened every day: At every inappropriate occasion he would touch her breasts or bottom to signalize his willingness for sexual interaction without caring at all about her being "in the mood" or not. This was hardly ever the case because she basically never felt she was being appreciated enough. He told her she had a sexual disorder and should see a professional. Sex is too important for him, he would otherwise leave her. By now she was doubtful herself, so that first she wanted to find out whether she was "really disturbed" or

> "still normal". Further treatment took place with involvement of the husband,
> followed by a couple therapy (see Chap. 6.1).

The higher prevalence of hypoactive sexual desire disorders in women indicates—
in the sense of the statistical "gender-typical" behavior—a stronger integration of
female sexuality into the entirety of (everyday) life and partnership quality and a
higher tendency of disturbance resulting from this. Female sexual behavior varies,
so, in each single case it needs to be investigated into, exactly what it is, that this
particular woman does not desire, does not find attracting. Furthermore, it should
be taken into account in which way generally an image of trivialized, brutalized,
commercialized relationship-lacking "sex" in today's "fun society" does not offer the
best conditions for the development and fulfillment of female sexuality. Presumably,
the new generation of adolescents come into contact with sexual erotic material
(pornography) and sexual violence (toward women) much too early and on the other
hand may not be familiar with affection and partnership comfort at all (see Chap. 7.1).

This also applies for the phase of hormone adjustment during menopause, which
is sometimes welcomed and used as an excuse for putting an end to an uncomfortable
sexuality. If, however, as in the case of bilateral ovarectomy, radiological, or chemo
therapy, there is abrupt hormone loss, hormone substitution is indicated.

Obviously, general physical condition, current diseases and the effects of their
medication therapy as well as possibly persistent hyperprolactinemia have to be
checked; however, in hypoactive sexual desire disorders, primary somatic causes,
e.g., pituitary-hypothalamic processes, are rare.

4.1.2   Disorders of Sexual Arousal

> Disorders of sexual arousal (ICD-10: F 52.2: DSM-IV-TR: 302,72) are diag-
> nosed when no arousal can be brought about despite the existence of sexual
> desire and physically adequate stimulation, meaning no or no complete erec-
> tion in males or rather no hyperemia (lubrication) of perivaginal tissue and
> labia in females.

Genital hyperemia normally makes penis penetration easier, i.e., lubrication of the
vagina enhances gliding capability and by the swelling up of the labia and the
so-called orgastic swelling friction with the penis. Lack of lubrication can cause
pain during intercourse, up to dyspareunia. Intravaginally measured values of vaginal bloodflow show that changes take place there even before being consciously
aware of "sexual arousal" and apparently vegetatively work even under traumatizing
circumstances.

The prevalence of erectile disorder has been well examined. In 17 % of the 40–70-year-old men questioned, the Massachusetts Male Aging Study (MMAS) established a minimal, in 25 % a moderate, and in 10 %, a complete failure of erection (Feldman et al. 1994). Braun et al. (2000) found erectile dysfunction in 19.2 % of their 4,489 more than 30-year-old respondents, in whom the authors were able to show that absolutely not all test persons with reported erectile dysfunction were unsatisfied with their sexual life.

Here, as well as in the frequency of dysfunctions, there was a significant age effect. The same is true for the Berlin Male Study (see Schäfer et al. 2003; Englert et al. 2007), in which the authors support the idea of differentiating between "erectile dysfunction" and "erectile disorder". In their opinion, only an "erectile disorder" is to be regarded as a pathological disorder, because the diagnosis is made according to DSM-IV-TR only if the disturbance causes "marked distress or interpersonal difficulty". An important finding in these surveys was the high coincidence between general medical symptoms (especially diabetes, heart disease, and high blood pressure). It is often overlooked that the occurrence of an erectile disorder beyond the age of 40 can be a first indication for chronic ischemic coronary disease (see Görge et al. 2003; Chew et al. 2008).

For most affected men, the first time of failing erection is indeed a drastic and shocking experience, putting their own "masculinity" at stake. In response to that, other (e.g., partnership) problems may be erroneously related to that fact. So, next to having an eye on function performance (by, e.g., prescribing PDE inhibitors) therapy is called upon to make the experience happen that successful intimacy is not inevitably dependant on erection capability.

> The "good news" reported in the interview study by Kleinplatz and Menard (2007) concerning people in long-term relationships (see Chap. 3.3): An intact erectile function is *not necessary* for successful sexuality.
>
> The "bad news", however, is: An intact erectile function is *not sufficient* for successful sexuality.

In addition, the overlapping of the dimension of reproduction has to be considered as potential interference, particularly in the case of involuntary childlessness, when the sexual experiencing of one or both partners is so dominated by the reproductive problem that uninhibited sexual contact does not seem possible any more.

> **Case Report 3** Two professional musicians in their late thirties (he a pianist, she a singer) had married 3 years before and saw their real calling in music, not necessarily aiming at mutual musical sessions and concert activities, but they did occur occasionally. Both their daily routine was marked by practice, travel, and concerts—often including phases of separation for weeks. Both had meanwhile developed a wish to establish a family and had not used contraceptives

for more than a year. Now, in the husband a situational erectile disorder had developed—both were despairing, pressure was extremely high, particularly because the wife reacted with blame.

The taking of various PDE-5 inhibitors in high doses had brought no improvement to the erectile function.

(for sexual therapy design see Chap. 6.3).

Again, the diagnostic and therapeutic approach of sexual medicine toward arousal disorders is marked by *"as well as"*. It is about acclaiming a new understanding of meaning concerning the dimensions of desire and attachment *as well as* applying the use of medication to improve sexual function. Clinical experience has shown that using only one of these paths exclusively has, in most cases, not helped the patient/couple to solve their problems. For this integrative approach, the current availability of different PDE-5 inhibitors for treatment of erectile disorders (but also of serotonin reuptake inhibitors for treatment of premature orgasm, see Chap. 4.1.3) means a major advance in the therapy of sexual disorders. For ideological reasons, however, these are neither meant to be used as an exclusive treatment option (this is a danger among the strictly somatic-orientated colleagues) nor as a generally excluded therapy option (a danger among the more psycho-therapeutically orientated colleagues).

Table 6.1 gives an overview of the various somatic treatment options (see Chap. 6.4).

As in the male equivalent, the *erectile disorder*, also in females the *arousal disorder* can develop into a vicious circle of anxiously apprehensive self-observation and concentration focusing on genital function, instead of heading toward a "mutual thing", making spontaneous build-up of arousal quite difficult.

The *syndyastic focus* (see Chap. 6.2.2) on experiencing intimacy while at the same time improving communication enables sexual arousal to develop without the encumbrance of anxious self-observation. At the same time, the partner is a part of the fundamental issue of being able to experience mutual intimacy in a playful, timeless, and sexually physical (body-talking) way, instead of working (alone) toward a quick coital feeling of satisfaction.

Case Report 4 The attractive 32-year-old (female) manager had been in a relationship for 1 year with a lawyer, 4 years older, and complained about lacking build-up of arousal in sexual interaction which now causes pain during vaginal intercourse resulting in her having "little desire for sex". Building up of arousal as well as achieving orgasm during masturbation was no problem.

The involved partner exclaimed to "go crazy", because nobody has such a "beautiful woman" at his side and he is nearly "dying with desire", while she is hardly to be activated—having, for example, had no sex at all during a holiday "on a tropical island".

The sexological assessment of the sexual preference structure of the woman revealed a complex sadistic pattern, which was vehemently rejected by her inner self: her arousal-increasing fantasies concerned torturing young men who are tied up and defenseless and are forced to perform involuntary sexual acts (for instance, performing cunnilungus). Vaginal penetration was never a part of her arousal-increasing fantasies. Again, in this case the couple-involving intervention proved itself by making the couple conscious of the immutability of sexual structure, understanding the pattern of her particular structure and at the same time still mobilizing resources of the partnership (see Chap. 6.3).

4.1.3 Disorders of Orgasm

Disorders of orgasm in men and women are different. In males, they mainly concern the point of time of orgasm ("premature ejaculation") and in females the difficulty of accomplishment or the lack of orgasm.

The following disorder categories are coded in the internationally relevant classification systems:

Premature orgasm (ICD-10: F 52.4; DSM-IV-TR: 302.75),
Delayed orgasm (ICD-10: F 52.3; DSM-IV-TR: 302.74), and
Missing orgasm (ICD-10: F 52.3; DSM-IV-TR: 302.73)

"Premature ejaculation" (in fact premature orgasm), defined as a constant occurrence of the climax before or immediately after penetration, over which the patient has no or very little control and is unable to experience a fully satisfying orgasm, is the most frequent sexual disorder in men. Approximately 20–25 % of men questioned in modern industrial countries have premature orgasm accompanied by psychological stress (Mathers et al. 2007; Porst et al. 2007). In giving valid prevailing figures, however, two problems arise: First, the normal ejaculation or orgasm time period is assessed highly subjectively and underlies great interindividual and also cultural variabilities (Althoff 2006; Montorsi 2005); secondly, exactly at this point it becomes obvious that "impairment of function" and clinically relevant disorders are not identical or concurrent (see Chap. 4.1).

Regarding the pharmaceutical options it is worth noting the results of clinical studies concerning Duloxetin (brand name Priligy), a serotonin reuptake inhibitor, which has now been released for the indication "orgasm praecox". Data show significant prolongation of the time period up to climax compared with the placebo-group. It was interesting to see that this group, taking the placebo substance, also reported a prolongation of the time period up to climax, but not as distinct as in the verum group (McMahon et al. 2008; Kaufmann et al. 2009).

Indeed, the general question about how objective these reports about phase prolongation remains (which, by the way, applies to all participants of the study); however, the data seems to verify the influence of serotonin for the neurophysiological relay of orgasm and can definitely be put to use in therapy. On the other hand, there is very likely a—probably small—group of patients who would benefit extremely, because in these patients the amounts of neurotransmitters which are provided by the synapses or the receptor itself have deficits. In most affected patients, however, there will presumably be regular conditions, which make the benefit from a serotonin reuptake inhibitor by far more subtle. Besides, in this case, as in all cases of sexual function disorder, there are presumably prevailing disturbances caused by partnership discontentment to be looked into and considered. This would explain, why "automatically" prescribed serotonin reuptake inhibitors for men with premature orgasm very often do not show the desired results.

Case Report 5 The first meeting with the 34-year-old tax consultant goes back to the year 1999, when he—at that time married for 8 years and father of two children aged 4 and 6 years—consulted the sexological out-patient department complaining of premature orgasm. His reported problem was primary and situational. Assessment revealed the typical stress situation during intimate contact with his wife, resulting from anxiety concerning recurrence of premature climax again. The wife, too, regretted this situation and he assumed she would be prepared to join a couple consultation. But it never came to that: neither the patient's wife nor the patient himself called again at that time.

Ten years later, the same patient showed up again with exactly the same problem, which had changed in no way at all over the years (in the meantime, however, he was father of four children). His wife was still dissatisfied with their sexual interactions and his taking serotonin reuptake inhibitors prescribed by the urologist to prolong the time span up to orgasm had not been successful, either.

Now, finally talking to the wife, it soon became obvious that she, since the birth of the children, had not felt satisfied about the interfamilial responsibility sharing and felt resentment about the fact that she had put her vocational interests behind for the sake of family management without gratification return concerning her own wishes and needs. After all, it was her husband who had the premature orgasm, so why should she take part in the therapy. Indeed, she was already missing out on so much, making sacrifices for the family, so she was not prepared to make any big efforts during sex, which she associated with relaxation and well-being.

Apart from the fact that this attitude increased the pressure on the husband, the real reason for her lacking willingness of cooperation was rooted in a chronically frustrated partnership contentedness—the unbearable and ever-present feeling of being taken for granted and taken advantage of.

Without therapeutic influence on this problematic topic, it would not be realistic to assume that the husband's sexual function disorder would be curable. Even with a medication-enhanced prolonged time phase to climax it would be predictable, that other aspects of contact arrangements would cause her grief and would most likely lead to other symptoms (e.g., erectile disorder).

From a sexological point of view this was an indication for a sexual therapy with a successful outlook, if both partners strive for improvement of their sexual contentedness and are prepared to go for this goal as a couple.

Causally, there could be a combination of somatic (e.g., short frenulum of the prepuce, balanitis) and psychosocial factors, considering the important part played by anxiety, insecurity, and pressure to perform (bearing in mind "masculinity myths"; see Zilbergeld 1994). Their origins could be on the individual and/or partnership level or could have their negative impact there.

Hypoorgasmia or anorgasmia in women is diagnosed, when orgasm is seldom or never reached, despite the existence of libido and adequate physical stimulation (clitoral, vaginal, breast stimulation, fantasies).

The prevalence of orgasm disorders (such as arousal disorders) has decreased over the past decades, from 80 % in the 1970s to 29 % in the 1990s of the last century, as shown in a study by Schmidt (1996), but is second place behind hypoactive sexual desire disorders when looking at female sexual disorders.

Many aspects affecting orgasm disorders have already been mentioned in connection with hypoactive sexual desire disorders and arousal disorders and do not have to be repeated. The great variety of erogenous zones, sexual stimuli and the range of reaction of women has been discussed and it has been pointed out that the partner has to be conscious of these differences (including the significance of teasing, petting, caressing, kissing, touching, etc.) in their double meaning on the orgastic and on the relationship level. Thus, hitherto-held distinctions in fore- and after-play become obsolete.

Different from male identity development, where exalting orgastic experience normally from the first ejaculation on hits on every time, females need to be aware of all of their erogenous zones and that orgasm may occur in their pubococcygeus muscle starting at the base of the spine and that they can also experience multiple orgasms. The female orgasm is learned during time or is discovered more or less accidentally and "practiced" in masturbation.

Once fixation on a particular autoerotic behavior is manifest, orgasm can be reached by masturbation but not during coitus. While in men sexual satisfaction and orgasm/ejaculation are generally synonymous, in females satisfaction and orgasm can be dissociated: postcoital total contentedness and satisfaction can be reached without orgasm, as well as a disturbed condition may prevail despite orgasm, depending on the quality of the partnership and the erotic acceptance of the partner. Experiencing intimacy, closeness, and security as well as feeling desired and simultaneously respected—in summary the fulfillment of elementary needs as a basis for sexual communication—can have more positive impact than experiencing orgasm. Still, in the long run, lack of orgasm will be regarded as a deficit with all the negative consequences of feeling inadequate as a woman. For that reason, and also to give the partner the feeling of being a good lover, orgasm is often faked. This, however, may lead to intrapsychic tension and—in the moment of truth—to a shock to the partner, in fact, the partnership itself.

As long as the prevailing orgasm disorder is not based on profound, elsewhere rooted disorders (possibly necessitating particular psycho-therapeutic treatment) sexual therapy will not dwell on the functional level, but will work on the issue of partnership and the significance of sexuality within this context. Here, refinement and enhancement of sexual stimulation strategies could be of great assistance.

Again, this involves the elementary needs, the communicative function of sexuality and the combination of genital and partnership pleasures. Then, taking one step at a time, working out their own particular likings, the couple can actually live through "new experiences" they had thought through together beforehand. As already pointed out in connection with disorders of arousal, in this way not only the partnership will be revived through more mutuality, frankness, and trust; also the focus of attention is turned *away from* self-observation, insecurity, performance pressure, and anxiety of failure *toward* a new view on the partner and the mutual intimacy, which exists completely independent of occurring orgasm, but due to the fixation on orgasm is not consciously perceived: Thus, the other important "climax", i.e., being unique and having been chosen by this particular partner, would remain unnoticed. It is this sense of belonging, however, which constitutes the healthy and/or healing bond of reliable partnerships. Particularly in times of numerous disappointed partnership experiences, the liberation, and strengthening of this salutogenic potential is a highly relevant goal of therapy. When this goal is anywhere near being reached, the probability of spontaneously reached orgasm experiences increases.

4.1.4 Dyspareunia

Both men and women can suffer from dyspareunia (ICD-10: F 52.6; DSM-IV-TR: 302.76). In men, however, it is rather seldom, which is why the issue here is mainly dyspareunia in women.

The expressions dyspareunia and algopareunia stand for the event of pain arising in connection with the penetration by the penis during sexual intercourse,
differentiated into disorder from the first coitus on (lifelong type), developed
after some period of no pain during intercourse (acquired type), occurring every
time (generalized) or only occurring under certain circumstances (situational).

Although dyspareunia has to be understood as a biopsychosocial entirety, the somatic
conditions must be looked into first of all. Only careful differentiating assessment
concerning the kind of pain, the place and time of occurrence during coitus or the
coital movements can indicate possible causes, e.g., inflammations, results of injuries
(during coitus, birth, accidents) or caused by operations with adhesions and scar
formation, atrophies, abnormalities, tumors, or endometriosis. The pain has its own
psychological effect on partnership comfort, so there is a possibility that it might not
disappear, even after the elimination of the main organic cause. In many cases, no
organic changes, which might explain the symptoms, are to be found, although the
(female) patients tend to look for physical causes. Probatory surgical interventions
are contraindicated, because these would support fixation on an organic cause and
in itself lead to new scar tissue or adhesions, etc. or tend to steer diagnosis into that
direction once more.

The obvious relevance of somatic factors causing development and maintenance
of dyspareunia is underlined by reports derived from larger clinical samples (see
Mendling 2008). In order to tackle the symptoms, many methods such as local anesthetics, local estrogens, or corticoids, tricyclic antidepressants, selective serotonin
reuptake inhibitors, injections of clonidine (to stimulate the alpha receptors) into
the vulva-accommodating peridural space as well as blockades of sympathic pre-
ganglionic nerve cells by injecting local anesthetics have been tried out—with as
little success as in employment of laser therapy. Also to be mentioned are therapeutic attempts with the calcineurine antagonists pimecrolimus and tacrolimus and the
anticonvulsive substance Gabapentin. Mendling (2008) mentions two new therapy
options which are not authorized on the German market for this indication, but might
be promising:

1. Botulinus toxin which blocks the peripheral acetylcholine release at the presynap-
   tic nerve endings for a number of weeks, thus causing muscle relaxation, which
   can be applied for various indications, e.g., in cases of hyper reagibility of the
   musculus detrusor in the field of urology (Schuch 2007). Gerber et al (2006) also
   report on Botulinus toxin A-injections (Botox) into the vulva muscle (20–40 mμE
   once or twice). The side effects resulting from this dosage are disregardably minor
   and the effect usually remained for 12 months.
2. Neocutis Bio-restorative Skin Cream (Neocutis S.A. Switzerland/San Francisco)
   which contains a lysate of cultivated cells with antiinflammatory cytokines. This
   cream is only available by prescription and is used dermatologically for improving
   scar tissue and is used in the USA as a skin care product. Gerber et al (2006) had
   61 women with "vulva vestibulitis syndrome" (average age 26 years, average

duration of illness 3 years) apply the cream twice daily with following results: No side effects were reported, 61 % described themselves as "healed", 33 % reported a much better, and 7 % a better sexual life.

Again it is apparent, that a therapeutic approach aiming solely at the somatic cause is characterized by the fact that the partner is not involved, which not only leads to losing important information about possible factors maintaining disorder within the partner relationship, but the relationship itself as a curative factor in the complete therapy is not made use of. Therefore, again, it needs to be stressed that *"as well as"* is more helpful for the patient/the couple than *"either—or"*.

Case Report 6 A 35-year-old female teacher has been married for 5 years to an architect of her own age and complains of a lifelong type of dyspareunia (first sexual intercourse at the age of 16, the symptoms prevailing for 19 years) and about "countless visits to gynecologists, not helping at all". Her current female gynecologist had recommended "a try at the department for sexual medicine". She, herself, was "completely sure" of some physical cause of her symptoms, the medical field has just not been able to find this cause and cure it.

She wants to have a "Botox-Injection" which she has read about and hopes to find relief this way. Her husband is being "very understanding". She wonders, "why he has not yet left me". The interview revealed massive expectation anxiety concerning the taking-up of sexual contact, the initiative has always been the husband's part, even though he—according to her report—is extremely cautious and would "rather do without it" than inflict pain on her.

This had led to a distinct reduction of coital contact to a maximum of once a month. Other sexual forms of interaction would take place now and then—bottom line being that she, as well as her husband both want to experience coital intimacy (exploration of her sexual preference structure revealed orientation to the adult male body scheme and exclusively vaginal-penetrative practice, which she would fantasize during masturbation leading to climax approximately once a month). Remarkable was her lacking readiness for the involvement of her partner into the diagnostic process. In the end she consented, having understood that this did not mean she could not have the favored "Botox-Injections". Furthermore, she agreed that the effectiveness of all measures and their sustainability can possibly be increased when all participants can be sure of support from their spouses.

Due to the fact that libido and/or lack of arousal, accompanied by failing lubrication, can cause complaints and could, in fact, lead to a dyspareunia, this could be the last link in a long chain of suffering. This is why all (like in orgasm disorders) before-mentioned factors and also therapeutic strategies are relevant here, because "life and partnership pains" can, in the sense of psychosomatic expression, appear as symptoms in the genital area and feign organic causes. The dividing line to vaginism can be blurred.

4.1.5   Vaginism

In fully developed vaginism (ICD-10: F 52.5; DSM-IV-TR: 306.51), the vagina is inaccessible and the gynecologist cannot examine the usual way, either. By any attempt of penetration (even just trying to insert a tampon) a (painless) reflex-like spasm of the distal third part of the vagina, the pelvis floor, and in some cases the adductor muscles of the thighs occurs. The patient is not even able to insert her own finger. In the pathogenesis of vaginism, biological ignorance, or wrong ideas (e.g., concerning anatomy, size, and elasticity of the vagina or the penis), irrational anxieties, myths, or own traumatizing experiences could play a role; in secondary vaginism, there could be partnership problems and rejection of the partner. Usually, the other sexual reactions are not disturbed, so that all sexual activity is possible, except for vaginal penetration. It might take years before help is sought for and even then the initiative often comes from the outside (e.g., their own parents want grandchildren) and not because of psychological distress. The partners of women suffering from vaginism are generally strikingly patient, understanding and considerate, and do not press the partner for changes. Such arrangements could be in the interests of both sides, for instance, the usually unpopular contraception issue is obsolete and the woman does not have to fear pregnancy and birth. The man does not have to worry concerning her fidelity and his potency, vocational goals can be aimed at, etc., all this remaining at a subconscious level.

The treatment demands great patience of both patient and counselor. A "penetrating" kind of therapy only makes things worse, not to mention such malpractice as vaginal dilations under anesthesia or surgical widening of the vaginal entrance. New experiences should be aimed at: The woman should try at being able to painlessly insert objects (increasing in size) harmlessly into the vagina in a relaxed position without panic, e.g., the so-called "Hegar's dilators" of increasing size or own fingers or a partner's finger up to insertion of the erected penis. If the woman kneels astride on top of the passive man, she herself is able to take control concerning the way and extent of penetration and is in a good position of getting over her (irrational) anxieties more easily. The individual experiences made by both partners, including possibly arising new problems (e.g., erectile dysfunction) is discussed during accompanying therapy and integrated into the (new) dimension of meaning of sexual communication within the partnership. Thus, the hitherto in a noncoital way experienced positive emotions concerning affection and intimacy can be brought more consciously or with expanded meaning into the coital sexuality. If this accompanying holistic approach is not applied, the vaginism may successfully be "trained away", but is liable to cause a change of symptoms, e.g., a hypoactive sexual desire disorder.

Case Report 7   Since 6 months, the 24-year-old female shop assistant had been in a partnership with her new boyfriend, a 25-year-old soldier, when she came to the out-patient clinic with a lifelong type of vaginism. Her scepticism that her boyfriend would not see the necessity of taking part in a sexual therapy turned out to be unwarranted. Sexual interaction between the two was very lively and included all sorts of contact forms (manual and oral stimulation, anal penetration as well), except vaginal penetration. The boyfriend described himself as being very happy in this partnership and assured everyone that he would gladly contribute to the goal of being able to have vaginal sexual intercourse at some point; he did find it "strange" that it would not work. Speedy advances in therapy were made and after already 4 weeks vaginal penetration was possible. Both claim this to have come about quite "by coincidence", while stroking each other, she sitting over him "suddenly felt his penis in my vagina", without feeling pain or restrictions of any kind. She was, however, so alarmed by this that they interrupted the intercourse and did not dare to try again soon.

This incident, however, quite vividly displays that expectation anxiety led to a reflexive tension that relaxed at a point, when she felt no more need for anxiety—because at that stage of therapy they had an agreement of not doing any penetrative interaction.

4.2 Disorders of Sexual Development

This area deals with disorders surfacing in the context of somatosexual, psychosexual, and sociosexual development over the whole lifespan which interfere with the persons' sexual interaction abilities, even as far as making sexual contact altogether impossible for them. This is not or not completely classified as a code (particularly DSM-IV-TR) within the current international classification system, although clinically highly relevant. In detail this concerns:

- Disorders of sexual maturity ((ICD-10: F 66.0: DSM-IV-TR: 302.9),
- Disorders of sexual orientation (ICD-10: F 66.1; DSM-IV-TR: 302.9),
- Disorders of sexual identity (ICD-10: F 66.8; DSM-IV-TR: 302.9), and
- Disorders of sexual relationship (ICD-10: F 66.2; DSM-IV-TR: 302.9).

Often, these disorders lead to secondary symptoms of other mental or behavioral disorders, which may then become the pretext for visiting the practitioner, suppressing the original problem itself. It is believed that most sexual development disorders as they are remain unconsidered and are only treated on the (secondary) symptom level—often because the individual is unable to state knowingly that the difficulties originally (or also) are rooted in personal sexual development.

This is even more so the case if the problem is embedded in complete development delay (retardation, physical, and psychological development disorder). Mental retardation as a handicap does not alter the dependency on the fulfillment of the fundamental needs for acceptance etc. and therefore also for intimacy, sexual contact, and desire for a sexual relationship.

4.2.1   Disorders of Sexual Maturity

The category disorders of sexual maturity (ICD-10: F 66.0; DSM-IV-TR: 302.9) deals with psychosexual and sociosexual effects of delayed or undeveloped physical sexual maturity (e.g., pubertas tarda). In many cases, it causes disturbances of gender and sexual identity formation and finally leads to developmental delay on the psychosexual/sociosexual level; it results in retardation of sexual development and difficulties in taking up sexual contact with potential partners of one's own age.

Disorders of sexual maturity are especially serious when they manifest themselves as sexual assault on children, because in such a case an adult suffering from somatosexual, psychosexual, or sociosexual retardation is restricted in his capabilities of forming adequate sexual relationships with persons of his own age and, seeking substitute gratification, uses children to meet his needs (Beier et al. 2005).

Case Report 8 Discrepancy between somatosexual and psychosexual development:

17-year-old A.M., until then without any criminal record, had sexually abused a 13-year-old boy as well as this boy's 11-year-old brother within a time period of 6 months. A.M. had been friends with both boys for a long time (the parents were on friendly terms); the mentally retarded A.M. (IQ of 65; unknown etiology) reports that the events in question happened, because he was trying to explain to them what "masturbation" means; for this reason he had shown them his "dick", placed himself in front of them and "taken his dick in his hand". The victims reported that he continued an "up and down movement". This happened several times. The 11-year-old describes: "His dick got big and then something came out of it. He then told me to do that, too. I then did it to myself. But my dick did not get big and nothing came out, either." Eventually, A.M. suggested an expansion of the action when he asked the boys to put his penis into their mouths or to "lick" it; only when he tried to go through with anal intercourse did the boys reject him and told their parents all about it, which led to charges against A.M.

During the exploration in the wake of an expert appraisal concerning the criminal responsibility, A.M. reported that he had had his first seminal discharge at the age of 13 and had since then regularly (once a week) masturbated, fantasizing exclusively sexual contact to girls of his own age or even older. He had no idea what a vagina looked like. The female body shape, especially the breasts of a grown woman, were very attractive to him. Furthermore, it did not escape him, that his 2 years older (not handicapped) sister was in intimate contact with her boyfriend, going as far as sexual intercourse. He himself had not been able to find an appropriate girlfriend of his own age yet. In fact, on the contrary, he had hardly dared to draw attention to himself, even in front of younger girls. Furthermore, he had no friends his own age—not earlier at the school for the handicapped nor now at the workshop for the handicapped. He therefore chose the company of younger children, whom he knew through friends of his parents; among these were the two victim boys. Concerning the sexual abuse A.M. is quite embarrassed, owns up to the offences and declares that he knows now that he should not have done these things. The parents were quite distressed about what had happened. They had been closely accompanying his development and had always been there for him. Due to the fact that he was a late-developer, they had not been prepared for him to have sexual needs "so early".

During the forensic evaluation it was taken for a fact that A.M.'s established physical sexual maturity had overtaken his psychomental maturity state. Only in contact with young children did he feel secure and respected, which was no problem at all, until—at the new stage of physical development—sexual needs arose that could not be dealt with adequately by children of that age. Therefore, with the onset of puberty at the age of 13 a strongly emotional destabilization concerning contact behavior took place: He felt drawn toward girls of his own age, but he lacked contact strategies, so that things remained at a certain point of tension (which the parents were not aware of). This explains the motivational background for the sexual abuse actions with the boys he had known and trusted for a long time. He "employed" them, so to speak, as an "experimental field" for fulfillment of his own needs for gathering sociosexual experience.

The offences are to be rated as a misplaced psychological processing of a "normal" physical development modus during age-appropriate puberty. Therefore, A.M.—due to his mental retardation—displayed lacking psychosocial competence compared with his peers (by whom he had not felt accepted) and had therefore very poor preconditions to cope with a "normal" adolescence crisis.

4.2.2 Disorders of Sexual Orientation

Sexual orientation toward one or the other gender is an axis of the human sexual preference structure, regardless of which type (homosexual, bisexual, or heterosexual) and is not to be defined as pathological or any kind of disorder, rather as a possible variation of human sexuality (see Chap. 4).

Apart from that, a problematic or pathological disorder of sexual orientation (ICD-10: F 66.1; DSM-IV-TR: 302.9) may develop, when a conflict in processing strategies and inadequate integration of the preferred orientation takes place, causing the person to suffer.

The individuals concerned feel burdened by the fact that—after completion of adolescence—they do not know whether or not they are orientated on the same gender. This uncertainty leads to incapability of social contact without anxiety or stress, because the conflict concerning the own sexual orientation obtains such a high level of importance, that all emotions, thoughts, and feelings are controlled by it. It culminates in brooding over the question of sexual orientation and fear that others could speculate about this issue or might allegedly identify whatever kind of sinister sexual orientation there might be.

The most frequent manifestation of sexual orientation disorder is to be found in homosexual orientation experienced as alien to one's self (the so-called "ego-dystone homosexuality"). At least, in the light of a sociocultural background of a heterosexual population majority, there are fears of actually being homosexual or of being unable to accept a realistic awareness of one's own homosexuality and certainly of not being able to integrate it into one's own sexual identity. Consequently, denial or suppression attempts follow which are usually of short duration and often lead to outright rejection of one's own sexual orientation: The result is a desire to change this condition. Not seldomly, relationships to the other gender are taken on, but these (some even with "technically" functioning sexuality) often do not work out due to lacking compatibility of sexual structure, remaining without real emotional indulgence on both sides. In the worst case, they end with a complete social and sociosexual withdrawal, resulting in isolation and loneliness and especially in psychoemotional deprivation—at a high risk of developing other mental or psychosomatic disorders. Therefore, the treatment obviously aims at an integration of the sexual orientation (not changeable anyway) into the own sexual identity and the whole self-concept of the person concerned (see Chap. 4.2.3).

Homosexual Orientation as a Problem in Medical Practice
Even, if at least in expert opinion, the knowledge should have been established by now that homosexual orientation is a normal variant of human sexuality and capacity for love. Due to a tradition over the centuries of pathologization and criminalization, the individuals themselves do often have considerable problems, usually starting at adolescence and requiring specialized (sexological) consulting skills. The *coming out*, meaning the development from the first moment of suspecting to be "different from the rest" up to the accepted certainty of being sexually orientated toward the same gender (homosexual) is—despite risen approval in society—sometimes still a painful process. Professionals should therefore lead adolescents to find *their individual* sexual

orientation and to help them accept it and integrate it into their personality. Most of all, it is the task of the consultant to locate the origin of anxieties concerning homosexual orientation and to invalidate these by talking and explaining.

Particularly in adolescents, it is greatly advised to also offer counseling to the parents (Lautmann 1995). Very often, worries concerning the future of their child are revealed and (sometimes massive) self-reproaches for "having done something wrong". Conveying an easily understandable biopsychosocial model of sexual orientation (this applies to homosexuality and heterosexuality alike), based on the concept of a broad variability of human sexuality is helpful here (see Bosinski 1992), as well as contact initiation to parent support groups for gay/lesbian adolescents.

Even for adolescents with heterosexual orientation, a sustainable relationship to the primary family based on acceptance and tolerance is an extremely important asset for successful blending in into the world of the "grown-ups"; it can be of surviving significance for adolescents in a situation of gay or lesbian coming out: If a feeling of "being different", being discriminated against and having difficulties in finding adequate partners—for exclusively homosexual individuals alone for statistical reasons understandably difficult—is additionally burdened by being left alone, this attitude contributes to high suicide rates in adolescents during homosexual coming out situations.

It needs to be conveyed to the adolescent (and often particularly to his or her parents) that homosexual orientation is a normal variant of human sexuality and capacity of love, totally compatible with an undisturbed identification with the gender of birth, that any kind of "reversion" is neither ethically justifiable nor possible and by no means necessary.

4.2.3 Disorders of Sexual Identity

A disorder of sexual identity (ICD-10: F 6.8; DSM-IV-TR: 302.9) is defined as an uncertain approach toward one's masculinity or femininity without questioning affiliation to one's own birth gender.

If gender identity is expressed by the question: "Am I a man or am I a woman?", then sexual identity is expressed by the question: "Am I a real male or a real female, i.e. sufficiently male or female?" So, it is all about feelings of adequacy and whether or not affected persons judge themselves as being a real man or a real woman, particularly in the sense of sexual attractivity, however that might individually be defined.

While in gender identity sexual attractivity does not play a leading part, in sexual identity the question arises whether one's own gender-typical qualities can be integrated into a sexual self-concept and whether gender-typical sexual behavior can be put into practice (see Diamond 2002).

In this context, mainly concepts and needs (allegedly) deviating from stereotype gender roles are relevant, particularly when they impress as unchangeable components of the sexual preference structure, but as such are not adequately perceived. This concerns especially the "third axis" of sexual preference structure, namely the manner of the favored sexual practice with the desired partner (see Chap. 4.4). If, in a man sexually orientated toward women, these are not directed at vaginal penetration, instead, for instance, a female foot has received fetish allocation (see the case report in Chap. 4.1), this might tend to a feeling of "not being a real man", because of repeated observation, not to come up to the expectations of the female sexual partner. Usually this is measured in comparison to what the concerned man believes "women (allegedly) want".

Taking on substantial, continuous sexual relationships may be especially difficult for men suffering from strong self-doubts and fear of failure concerning their sexual performance and potency, triggering anxiety.

This is the case in "male identity disorder" with resulting consequences for self-evaluation and an inner attitude toward the male gender role, as well as toward trust in their own (sexual-) functional adequacy as a "man". This often is the basis for men wishing to alter physical features, such as breast (M. pectoralis) and buttock implants (M. glutaeus) and penis extensions. This development can be described as "sociosexual self-insecurity", which far exceeds general, i.e., surmountable "shyness in the face of the other sex" and can be one reason for affected persons remaining without desired partnerships over a long period of time.

Case Report 9   The 42-year-old pilot had had a circumcision done a year ago, even though vaginal intercourse (his favored sexual preference) was possible before without any problems and he had easily been able to reach climax. He had had countless short-termed partnerships and absences from home due to his profession were often additionally used for short sexual contacts to various women. It had always been important for him that his sex-partners should "get their money's worth" and "get as much from it, as him". The reason for the circumcision was the allegedly increasing insensitiveness during sexual intercourse which, from his point of view, led to a situation in which he was not able to experience the sexual contact with the usual relaxedness and this made him fear that his partners might "not be satisfied", even though he had not had any feed-backs along this line. He had hoped to reach a higher state of sensitivity of the glans penis by the circumcision, which did not turn out to be the case, this again makes him feel uncomfortable, because now he thinks, during sexual contact he will be "even more tense".

4.2.4 Disorders of Sexual Relationship

A disorder of sexual relationship is given, when the concerned individuals suffer from lacking sexual contentedness within their partnership and do not see any possibility of bringing about a change of the situation as a couple. Usually both partners are concerned and the cause for the lacking contentedness is a frustration of fundamental needs for acceptance and emotional security and the feeling of being important and right for each other.

Disorders of sexual relationship can be caused by other sexual disorders, such as disorders of sexual function: For example, an erectile disorder in a man or dyspareunia in a woman can easily lead to a feeling of not being able to live up to the expectations of the partner, not getting any esteem from the partner and not being worthy of these anyway. Seen from another angle, a disorder of sexual relationship can itself lead to a disorder of sexual function, for instance, because of lacking feelings of esteem by the partner, feelings of not being wanted by the partner, the willingness to indulge in sexual activity decreases, possibly resulting in the development of a disorder of sexual desire (see Chap. 4.1.1).

But also in sexual preference disorders (see Chap. 4.4) there is great danger, that the concerned individuals develop doubts (not quite unfounded) of still being accepted by the partner, if he/she knew the details concerning the peculiarity of the preferential inclination at hand. This, however, leaves the individual without the possibility of ever being sure of really being wanted by the partner, namely just the way he/she is, i.e., notwithstanding their particular sexual inclination.

On the other hand, it is always feared—were the truth about the sexual peculiarities known—that the partner would retreat and not wish to continue the partnership any more.

Disorders of sexual relationship are extremely common, but very seldomly diagnosed, although in many cases they present the background for reduced life quality and happiness.

The psychological stress arising from this condition is often a negative factor influencing life quality in general and health in particular. The reasons for these problems may well lie in the spectrum of other sexual disorders (see above), as well as in psychological and behavioral disorders, which make taking up and/or maintaining sexual relationships difficult or impossible.

In this context, attention should be paid to the curtailment of the syndyastic function level resulting from a not adequately integrated attachment dimension of sexuality.

If, for instance, the dimension of desire is separated from the dimension of attachment, this can result in an exaggeration of the dimension of desire at the expense of the attachment dimension, which is more often found in men than in women. These men are then so focused on pleasure and its satisfaction in sexual experience, that they do not experience this within the context of being connected with a partner relationship. Their partner often reacts by sexual withdrawal, because during sexual interaction they do not feel "personally appreciated and accepted" or even feel "abused".

This separation can also take place and even be favored by an exclusively pharmaceutical symptomatic treatment of erectile disorder (e.g., PDE-5-inhibitors) without therapeutic back-up and without involving the partner of the individual concerned and may cause (unintended) increase of sexual relationship disorder.

One reason why many men use erection-enhancing medication for only a short period of time—aside from the high costs—is because their partners signal that obviously the male's focus is on achieving erection and thus on the experience of lust, so that the women feel their own need for attachment, warmth and security is neglected and ignored—they feel disregarded and even degraded.

Also, if the dimension of reproduction is unbalanced, i.e., overemphasized, it can lead to a sexual disorder, for instance, when one partner aims at sexual contact only for reasons of reproduction, while perhaps the other partner does not share the strong desire for children and would refuse sexual intercourse. Often, a disorder of sexual relationship again expresses itself in the absence of sexual reactions, respectively in sexual dysfunctions, e.g., anorgasmia of the woman or even of the man (ejaculatory deficiency) during vaginal coitus.

4.3   Disorders of Gender Identity

Patients with this disorder show insecurities, irritation, and misperception concerning their own gender affiliation (ICD-10: F 64.0; DSM-IV-TR: 302.85). An inner sense of belonging to the other gender is dominant, contrary to their own biological birth gender. They feel that they are living in the "wrong" body and have a strong wish to change this situation.

Within this disorder group there are different levels and stages with varying causes and these must be dealt with in different ways. For this reason, these problems are summarized under the collective term *gender identity disorders*. A passing (not persistent) sense of discomfort in one's own gender, discontentment, and insecurity regarding one's own social gender role, cosmetic or other subjectively founded personal needs for measures to alter body contours have nothing whatsoever to do with this group. Persons with a genuine gender identity disorder nearly always need specialized psychotherapeutic treatment, the aim of therapy not being to "combat" or "reverse" the desire or to achieve a change in gender, but solely to offer these persons a strategy for tackling their own gender identity insecurity over a long period of time and with an open outcome. At the same time, therapeutic guidance allows the patient to test the gender genuinely felt under all circumstances and in all social areas of their own everyday life (the so-called "real-life test"). With skilled counseling and advice the patient will be able to understand and process the developing impressions, experiences, and feelings. Here, again, the relevance of the fundamental psychosocial needs has to be pointed out, because feeling accepted and not rejected concerning the ambivalent gender situation is of utmost importance for these persons in the context of professional care.

Accordingly, the most important differential diagnoses *during adolescence* are sexual maturity crises (see Chap. 4.2.1) on one hand or a repelled (suppressed or denied) not integrated homosexual orientation (see Chap. 4.2.2) on the other, or transvestitic fetishistic and autogynephilic preference disorders (see Chap. 4.4), serious personality disorders as well as—although more seldom—psychotic diseases. In adolescents, it takes diagnostic-therapeutic accompanying respectively sexological treatment with indeterminate outcome, allowing the concerned individuals to get to the bottom of their identification conflict. However, alongside the continuous verification of the wish to transform the gender, special attention should also be given to other developmental functions or conflicts beyond the problem of gender identity (Korte et al. 2008).

In biological adult men, transvestitic fetishism is one of the most important and frequent differential diagnoses (see Chap. 4.4); in biological women it is a not integrated (ego-dystonic) homosexual orientation. Moreover, personality disorders require particular attention. Complicating the assessment process, they may explain the problems of gender identity (e.g., a borderline personality disorder) but can also be found additionally.

In the interest of the patients it is therefore recommended, not to make any diagnosis before testing real-life conditions in the desired gender role under therapeutic guidance—in Germany for at least 1 year according to the "Standards of Treatment and Expert Assessment of Transsexuals" of the sexological societies (Becker et al. 1997)—in order to be quite sure of an enduring transsexual gender identity disorder (which is important for legal aspects as well; see Chap. 5.2.2) and then initiating proceedings for body-changing measures.

The strongest and irreversible form of gender identity disorder is described as *transsexuality*. In such rather seldom cases, the origin lies in a lifelong persisting conviction of an irreversible, i.e., final disintegration of one's own masculine or feminine body feeling (the conviction of living in the wrong body). As stated above, diagnosis can only be made in the course of time, when the concerned persons have lived of ordinary everyday life in their preferred gender role. After secured diagnosis these cases, showing "persistent, well documented gender dysphoria" (WPATH 2011), usually have to be treated with cross-gender hormone medication and in indicated cases with sex-reassignment surgery, along with the necessary psychotherapeutic sessions. In other cases of gender identity disorders (i.e. not meeting the above mentioned criteria), the priority is on psychotherapy accompanying attainment of a suitable identity, while body-altering measures (hormones, surgery) are usually not considered as being indicated (and therefore will not, like in Germany, be covered by the insurance system).

As transsexuality (i.e., the irreversible form of gender identity disorder) cannot be diagnosed before getting sufficient data on the individuals' psychosexual and somatosexual development (which consolidates through the influence of hormones), in adolescents the administration of medication used to block the process of puberty

(GnRH-Analoga) respectively cross-gender hormone medication can only be approved of in singular cases preceding careful proof by different experts. The critical point of maturity ascertainment and the resulting indication for hormonal intervention should therefore not be fixed depending on the age of a person, but bearing on the individual development in each singular case and it should always be done interdisciplinarily (de Vries and Cohen-Kettenis 2012).

There is no verified knowledge to date how hormonal treatment prior to completion of puberty might influence further development of gender identity. Therefore, even in a retrospectively successful treatment case, it may not inevitably be true that originally there was a definite transsexual determination in the first place.

A child or an adolescent is generally not equipped with the necessary emotional and cognitive maturity to consent to a treatment involving lifelong consequences. Therefore, it must be taken into consideration that children with gender identity disorder more than averagely show deficits of social competence, behavior deviations, and psychiatric comorbidities (see Wallien et al. 2007), which makes them particularly susceptible for the temptations of an allegedly "fast cure" concerning all their problems.

It is also necessary to keep in mind the huge range of the developmental trajectories of persistence and desistence of childhood gender dysphoria and the psychosexual outcome of gender dysphoric children, underlining the importance of their social environment, the first experiences of falling in love and sexual attraction, which could influence their gender-related interests and behavior as well as their feelings of gender discomfort and gender identification (Steensma et al. 2011). Data of a qualitative study carried out with 25 adolescents diagnosed with a gender identity disorder in childhood indicate that they considered the period between 10 and 13 years of age to be crucial for the persistence or desistence of their childhood dysphoria, underlining the importance of their social environment, the anticipated and actual feminization, or masculinization of their bodies, the first experiences of falling in love and sexual attraction had influenced their gender-related interests and behavior as well as their feelings of gender discomfort and gender identification (Steensma et al. 2011).

If criteria are given for the diagnosis of transsexuality, the cross-gender hormone treatment for feminization or masculinization must not be commenced before the patient has received detailed verbal and written explanation about the effects and side-effects of hormone treatment. In this context it must be made clear that hormone substitution is a lifelong option, necessary to avoid threatening hormonal deficiencies.

The application of cross-gender hormones leads to irreversible, i.e., only surgically correctable body changes (atrophia of the gonads and gynecomastia in biological men, hirsutism and breaking of the voice in biological women).

The idea that gender identity could in any way be strengthened by hormone application is wrong. This is true "for both directions", i.e., concerning the wrong belief that application of same gender hormones would strengthen the birth gender and thus "heal" gender identity disorder as well as concerning the wrong idea that cross-gender hormone replacement therapy would finally bring a vague gender identity disorder into the "clear form" of transsexuality. Specialized literature (Hembree et al. 2009) gives information on medical laboratory preexaminations and the course of measurements concerning cross-gender hormone treatment and the recommended substances (including dosages).

4.4 Disorders of Sexual Preference (Paraphilias)

Patients with *disorders of sexual preference (paraphilias)* experience deviating sexual impulses, which are a part of their sexual preference structure.

The sexual preference structure in general manifests itself in every human on three basic axes: (1) with regard to the preferred gender of the sex partner (male and/or female), (2) regarding the preferred (body development) age of the sex partner (body scheme of children, adolescents, adults, elderly persons), and (3) regarding the preferred kind and modus of sexual activity with and without sex partner(s) (type, object, method, etc.).

The final manifestation of sexual preference structure takes place during youth and remains a constituent for life in its basic features and is invariable. This includes invariability of particular sexual inclinations, which are also manifest from youth on and which partly or completely characterize the sexual structure of the person involved.

Exactly these individual manifestation forms on the three axes mentioned decide which stimuli sexually attract each individual, so that this alone would enable a huge spectrum of principally resulting possibilities. Important is, however, that the greatest intensity of pleasure attainment is to be reached by the personal arousal pattern, therefore this pattern essentially rules the sexual experience of each individual. But this also means that sexually stimulating signals differing from the personal arousal pattern are not prone to develop comparable intensity of pleasure—even when eagerly desired. A male, sexually orientated toward females (Axis 1), then toward the adult development shape (Axis 2), and in sexual interaction toward female feet (Axis 3), will never during coital intimacy with a woman experience the same intensity of pleasure as he would in giving attention to her feet, which could (considerably) differ from the sexual preference pattern of the real (female) partner.

From a sexological point of view, only such cases are diagnosed as disorders of sexual preference or paraphilia which cause the individual to suffer by his deviant sexual impulses.

Table 4.2 Disorders of sexual preference/paraphilias by ICD10/DSM-IV-TR

	ICD-10		DSM-IV-TR
F65.0	Fetishism	302.81	Fetishism
F65.1	Transvestic fetishism	302.3	Transvestic fetishism
F65.2	Exhibitionism	302.4	Exhibitionism
F65.3	Voyeurism	302.82	Voyeurism
F65.4	Pedophilia	302.2	Pedophilia
F65.5	Sadomasochism	302.83	Sexual masochism
302.84	Sexual sadism		
302.89	Frotteurism		
F65.6	Multiple disorders of sexual preference		
F65.8	Other disorders of sexual preference		
F65.9	Sexual disorder not otherwise specified	302.9	Not otherwise specified paraphilia

Therefore, persons who have such inclinations, but do not suffer by them, are not considered disturbed, ill, or in need of treatment, as long as they do not impair or endanger others or themselves by acting out their deviating sexual needs (Table 4.2).

First epidemiological data shows (Langström and Zucker 2005; Ahlers et al. 2008) that the prevalence of paraphilia-related sexual arousal patterns is higher than assumed. This is true for German-speaking countries based on data of the *Berlin Male Study (BMS)* in which the prevalence of erectile dysfunction, its age-dependency and its relation to general health variables as well as quality of life measures were determined in 6,000 men aged 40–79. In the first phase of this study 1,915 men took part (Schäfer et al. 2003). These men were then invited to take further part in a comprehensive sexological study by responding to an extensive questionnaire on sexual experiences and behavior, including their (female) partners (later also examined). The outcome was a sample of 373 men, of whom 63 were single and 310 involved in a relationship (108 female partners were additionally involved and personally interviewed). The data gives an impression of possible paraphilia-related tendencies within the general population by inquiring arousal patterns which were characterized according to frequency of occurrence in sexual fantasies, during masturbation (as contents of fantasies), and during actual practice (Ahlers et al. 2009).

Total 57.6 % of the questioned men recognized one of these arousal patterns as part of their fantasies, 46.9 % used them for arousal enhancement during masturbation, and 43.9 % acted out these patterns on the behavioral level. Even though the obligatory, almost unavoidable selection effects do not allow these figures to be applied to the general population, there is nevertheless a relevant indication given about the presumptive distribution, which explains the extent and diversity of offers from the pornography industry (Table 4.3).

It is, however, to be assumed that the most "deviating" sexual impulses are rooted in the "normal" sexual response and only turn into pathological disorders by their isolation or generalization.

The DSM-IV-TR (APA 2000) takes this into account by coding a diagnosis only if the involved person claims to suffer on account of this paraphilic inclination or if it causes restrictions in significant social or vocational life functions, or, if paraphilias potentially endanger others (e.g., a pedophilic inclination, regardless of any possible

Table 4.3 Prevalence of paraphilia-associated sexual-arousal patterns on different experience levels in men between 40 and 79 years (no clinical population-based sample); results of the Berlin male study II

Levels of experience	Sexual fantasies		Fantasies accompanying Masturbation		Sexual behavior	
	N	(%)	N	(%)	N	(%)
Nonhuman objects (e.g., material or shoes—fetishism)	110	29.5	97	26.0	90	24.1
Wearing female clothes (transvestic fetishism)	18	4.8	21	5.6	10	2.7
Being humiliated (masochism)	58	15.5	50	13.4	45	12.1
Torturing other persons (sadism)	80	21.4	73	19.6	57	15.3
Secretly watching others in intimate situations (voyeurism)	128	34.3	90	24.1	66	17.7
Presenting one's genitals to strangers (exhibitionism)	13	3.5	12	3.2	8	2.1
Touching strangers in public (frotteurism, toucheurism)	49	13.1	26	7.0	24	6.4
Childrens' bodies (pedophilia)	35	9.4	22	5.9	17	3.8
Not otherwise specified	23	6.2	23	6.2	17	4.6
Sexual response to at least one arousal pattern/stimulus	215	57.6	175	46.9	163	43.7

Responses for different arousal patterns were prompted on a 5-step rating-scale with gradings: -none, -few, -moderate, -strong, -very strong. All answers from "few" to "strong" were rated as a response to a sexual arousal pattern $N = 373$

distress of the inclined individual himself), as a result of the involved person having acted out his impulses.

On the basis of these findings it is quite remarkable that a significant number (nearly one-third) of the questioned men taking part in *BMS II* regarded paraphilia-related sexual arousal patterns as inadequate and voluntarily relinquished acting them out—even if these do not involve harming or endangering others (e.g., fetishistic impulses). Nonetheless, an also remarkable number of participants revealed a potential for sexual violation of self-determination of others (e.g., exhibitionism, voyeurism, frotteurism) or had already taken part in sexual (e.g., pedosexual) infringement in the past.

It is not seldom for different paraphilias to occur side by side; a great number of exceptional inclinations are known of, which, in the international classification systems, are summarized as "not otherwise specified paraphilias" or "other disorders of sexual preference" (Table 4.4).

Table 4.4 Selection of rare paraphilic sexual arousal patterns with erotic focus and possible overlapping with other paraphilias

Term for the paraphilia	Erotic focus	Possible overlapping with other paraphilias
Zoophilia	Animals	
Klysmaphilia	Clyster	Sexual masochism
Suffering or humiliation of oneself or the partner		
Obscene phone calls (telephone scatophilia)	Obscenities on the telephone	Exhibitionism
Salirophilia	Soiling or disheveling clothing or bodies	Sexual sadism
Partners not able to consent		
Necrophilia	Corpses	
Self-stimulation or stimulation of others with atypical objects		
Hypoxyphilia/asphyxia	Reduced oxygen intake	Sexual masochism
Morphophilia	Particularly pronounced physical characteristics in the partner	Partialism
Amputophilia	Amputations in the partner	Morphophilia, partialism
Apotemnophilia	Own amputation	Sexual masochism
Infantilism	Being treated as an infant	Sexual masochism, fetischism
Gerontophilia	Highly aged partner	
Autogynaephilia	Experiencing oneself as a woman without rejection of male genitals	Transvestitic fetischism
Urophilia, coprophilia	Urine, faeces	Fetischism, sexual masochism, sexual sadism
Vampirism, cannibalism	Human blood, flesh	Fetischism, sexual sadism

Particularly autogynephilia (Blanchard 1989) is clinically known as a sexual preference expressing a wide range of conditions with and without marked distress, also with and without effects on gender identity (Chap. 4.3).

There is further literature on diagnostic details and symptoms concerning these specific inclinations in Money (1986, 1989) and Beier (2007). However, it applies to all kinds of paraphilic experience, the common and the exceptional, that, according to all empirical data, these are a domain of male sexuality and can therefore—particularly during puberty of male adolescents—become relevant. Same applies to the development of pedophilic inclination (i.e., sexual attraction toward prepubescent body scheme, i.e., development stage before beginning growth of pubic hairs and breasts).

Hebephilia (i.e., sexual attraction toward early pubescent body scheme meaning development stage with beginning growth of pubic hairs and breasts etc., i.e. Tanner stages 2 and 3—while the sexual preference for the late male pubescent body scheme is called "ephebophilia" and for the late female adolescence "parthenophilia") is an independent disorder of sexual preference to be diagnosed according to the International Classification System of the World Health Organization (ICD-10) or the American Psychiatric Association (DSM-IV-TR), not yet specifically coded (for DSM-V there are plans to change this). In clinical work, however, this disorder plays an important role.

Sexual preference structure is of great significance concerning development of sexual identity, because the preference—beginning at the onset of puberty at the latest-controls the contact mode toward one's social circle and reference persons. It is therefore not at all trivial, whether the sexual impulses are adequately integrated into the self-image, resulting in a secure sexual identity, no matter how deviant. This already applies to acceptance of the own body and its genitals which is often difficult—particularly in personal comparison with protagonists supplied by media and internet pornography—even in the case of ordinary preference structure, the integration of which is always an additional developmental performance. Although first sexual self-confidence is generally built up by successful sociosexual experience, it is still plausible to consider the idea of disruptive elements in these developmental processes, particularly when it might be assumed that the (alleged) expectations of partners cannot be lived up to (see Chap. 7.1) or, in the case of paraphilic impulses, efforts of partnership contact "come to nothing" and thus lead to syndyastic deprivation. Under certain circumstances "disorder of sexual identity" may then result. This is defined as a recurrent and intense feeling of uncertainty concerning own male or female quality as a sexual partner (see Chap. 4.3). Due to the fact that the establishment of paraphilic impulse patterns during adolescence and their unchangeability makes it necessary for the individuals concerned to cope with these inner emotional issues during their development of sexual experience, they may be more or less heavily burdened with self-doubts. In the end, these result from the answer to the question whether a partner would completely accept them, if only the contents of their sexual fantasies were known—meaning, even if their achievement (with a partner) were not intended at all. This feeling of uncertainty touches syndyastic experience so significantly ("can I find real acceptance in the other?") that partnerships are hard to accomplish or existing partnerships are at high risk. This can be due to ignorance concerning the progression of paraphilic inclination (will it recede, remain the same or increase at some point?) or perhaps due to a situation of having to hide for years (shielding the paraphilic parts from the partner) which leads to more loss of trust if the inclination becomes disclosed by other circumstances (increasingly more disclosures of internet activities by the partner).

Case Report 10 Twenty-one-year-old patient with an exclusively masochistic sexual preference pattern.

The frail, highly intelligent student of engineering science came because of a primary situational orgasm disorder which had arisen time and time again since the first intimate contact with the 2 years older girlfriend in this, his first sociosexual relationship, now going on for 6 months. The assessment of sexual preference structure revealed an exclusively masochistic pattern with operation scenes, in which female doctors supported by OP nurses (never a man in sight) mutilated him and watched him suffer—also putting on a chastity belt in the operating theatre was an arousal-enhancing fantasy. This was meant to put painful pressure on the penis and prevent erection. The feeling caused by the bound chastity belt was simulated during masturbation by him lying on his stomach, holding his penis tightly in his hand in order to "press" the genital "to a maximum". Only in this way was he able to reach climax, not by vaginal penetration, for which the erection was strong enough, but did not create enough stimulation in order to reach orgasm. His girlfriend, later interviewed, reported that she had found him to be "completely tense" and was worried that he might be "gay".

Because both partners were authentically interested in a mutual perspective, a syndyastic sexual therapy was applied (cf. Beier and Loewit 2004), not aimed at changing the sexual preference structure, rather—after truthfully explaining the background problems of the patient—revealing to the partner his difficulties of sexual communication. In fact, the explanation concerning the connection to the paraphilic experience was a huge step for both partners during therapy. The goal of sexual therapy was to achieve unpreoccupied intimate communication. In the end, it was helpful that he did not have to be afraid of oncoming sexual arousal because the fantasies he has during that period were then not perceived as "deception of the girlfriend" any more.

As far as the goal of the therapeutic approach is concerned, the focus (as shown in the case history above) is on the existential level of the indispensable psychosocial fundamental needs, thus putting sexuality onto a larger scale of meaning, because it is all about the mutual fulfillment of these basic needs (syndyastic dimension) for both partners within their relationship.

This, exactly, is the reason why, in a disorder of sexual preference, i.e., paraphilia, the syndyastic focus is regarded to be an appropriate therapeutic strategy—as long as both partners are keen on improving their sexual and partnership relationship comfort, well aware of the necessary decrease of selfishness within the partnership. However, this can only be the case, if the paraphilic stimulus of the inner experience world of the individual concerned is not of greater importance than the attachment itself.

This shows that during diagnosis of paraphilia the exploration of the three dimensions (attachment, desire, and reproduction) should be regarded as an indispensable element, because by this the range of therapeutic choices and therewith linked chances of improvement become assessable (see Chap. 6.3).

4.5 Disorders of Sexual Behavior (Dissexuality)

This category summarizes all forms of sexual behavior by which health and well-being of others is damaged or their sexual self-determination is endangered. *Dissexuality* is defined as failure to conform to social norms—regardless of whether

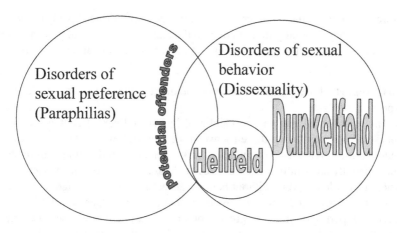

Fig. 4.4 Disorders of sexual preference and sexual behavior

that failure has been prosecuted or not. It concerns all harmful sexual conduct (physical or psychological violence) and is defined as irresponsible sexual behavior which disregards the individual rights of others (Beier 1995).

Attempts at or actual performance of sexual acts in front of, with or by prepubescent or pubescent minors or other persons unable to consent to these, also belong to the category of sexual behavior disorders (the so-called "pedo-sexual" acts; in criminal law: "sexual abuse of children (csa)").

Some cases of disorders of sexual behavior can be attributed to acting out certain paraphilias, i.e., a paraphilic impulse pattern (see Chap. 4.4) can be the root of disturbed sexual behavior, defined as *acts of inclination*. In other cases, dissexual behavior is related to a different primary, problem, e.g., personality disorder, mental retardation, low sociosexual experience as in some adolescents and—presumably most important of all—boundary-violating family constellations with generally unfavorable conditions of child development (see Chap. 7.3). Such cases of sexual abuse are (seen from the perspective of the offender) motivationally understood as *substitute acts,* compensating the actually desired sexual interaction with an adult and consenting partner, which for several reasons is not obtainable in a socially acceptable manner. For sexological diagnosis this implies that disorders of sexual preference and sexual behavior have to be well differentiated and not confused, or even equated.

In a diagram, Fig. 4.4 shows that within the whole spectrum of paraphilias the preponderant part has *nothing* to do with harmful sexual contact, i.e., dissexuality. Conversely, dissexuality is *usually not* attributed to paraphilia. In simple terms, the majority of men with disorders of sexual preference ("paraphilia") are not dissexual, and the large number of men with sexual behavior disorders ("dissexuality") are not paraphilic. Child sexual abuse (CSA) studies in the *Hellfeld* (legally registered cases) show that approximately 40 % of violations are assigned to pedophilically motivated offenders and 60 % to substitute acts (see Seto 2008).

Moreover, only a minor number of dissexual acts are performed openly (*Hellfeld*), meaning that they generally do not come to the attention of the courts or the police (*Dunkelfeld*)—but do, however, play an important role in clinical sexual medicine.

Case Report 11 Eighteen-year-old pedophile, orientated to boys, exclusive type.

The high-school graduate, no siblings, had staged sexual contact to pre-pubescent boys by luring these (between the age of 7 and 10 years) victims under various pretences into cellars or parks, demanding of them to stimulate him manually and orally; in some cases anal intercourse took place. Most offences (10 at least) went without being registered, until, at the age of 16, he was cautioned for the first time by a juvenile court and then, aged 18, rendered to expert opinion in the process of a criminal procedure. The things he actually did to these boys completely coincided with the fantasies accompanying masturbation, i.e., involving prepubescent boys who voluntarily carried out oral stimulation or who would let themselves be penetrated anally. This patient was clearly aware of his sexual orientation and he was certain—unlike his parents—that it was not going to change. In the course of the first criminal procedure, his father, in particular, had made efforts to employ different therapists who were supposed to help his son "to get something started with women". He told the expert witness that he would be prepared to give his son enough money so that he could visit prostitutes; he was sure his son was only "too shy" to have "normal sex" and was "absolutely certain" that no pedophilia was involved, in fact declared that "all pedophiles need to be executed".

This example illustrates the possible overlapping of sexual preference disorders with sexual behavior disorders, often arising during puberty and the great significance of environmental factors for an adequate access to the own problems: The concerned adolescent had hardly any chance of expecting understanding for his homo-pedophilic sexual orientation, although it had not been his own choice and could not be influenced. In such cases it is difficult to enforce primarily preventive measures aiming at recognizing the concerned individuals as soon as possible—best during their adolescence—in order to prepare them as early as possible for a responsible dealing with their inclination and to support them by suggesting coping skills options. In addition, in this context the influence of the internet and the new media (see Chap. 7.2) has to be particularly stressed, because experience in clinical work reveals direct connection between consumption of internet pornography or sexualized games contents on one hand and disorder of sexual behavior including sexually traumatizing acts on the other. One example concerning consenting sexual contact in adolescents would be sudden, pre-orgastic switching form vaginal penetration to oral sex by the young man, aiming at ejaculation into the face or the mouth of his young girl-friend. This so-called "cum-shot" is a stereotype feature of pornographic film sequences and is hardly ever missing at the end of any filmed sexual interaction, so that the adolescent may take it for granted that the young girl he just had sex with was longing for such a "cum-shot", just like the actress shown in the porn film was.

In fact, there are enough known cases in which the young (female) sexual partner did not want that at all, but was lacking experience and not superior enough during the actual intimate situation to react and resist.

Another example is the viewing of sexualized games, freely accessible on the internet, which can animate children to perform the shown procedures (e.g., oral intercourse) in reality.

In order to be able to assess disorders of sexual behavior in adolescents, it is, of course, necessary to acquire knowledge about the availability of pornographic offers on the internet and the various numerous freely accessible browser games, as well as about the different communication channels for adolescents on the internet (e.g., Facebook, Myspace, etc.) which function as forums for exchanging information.

4.6 Disorders of Sexual Reproduction

Disorders of sexual reproduction are characterized by psychological and psychophysiological impairment of reproduction in its various phases ([pre]conception, pregnancy, birth, as well as child care and raising); they cause significant suffering and/or difficulties within human relationships as well as endangering social integration. Adequate coding by the current international classification systems (ICD-10 and DSM-IV-TR) is not possible, but needed urgently. From a clinical point of view, however, they are indeed distinguishable (see Beier et al. 2006):

- *Preconceptional disorders:* For example, involuntary childlessness; pseudocyesis (imagined pregnancy): In such cases, nonexisting physical and psychophysiological conversion processes normally assigned to a manifest pregnancy (suspended menstruation, weight gain, striae, lactation, child movement) are actually experienced by the woman and presented convincingly to her social environment.
- *Prenatal disorders:* For example, denied pregnancy: In such cases, physical and psychophysiological conversion processes normally assigned to a manifest pregnancy (suspended menstruation, weight gain, child movement) are not perceived by the pregnant woman (negated) or are hidden from the perception of others (concealed); furthermore, abortions and miscarriages belong to this category.
- *Postnatal disorders:* For example, postpartal depression, certain characteristics in educational behavior such as child neglect or maltreatment, but also treating the child as a self-object (see Beier 1994; Beier et al. 2005).

Case Report 12 Not perceived pregnancy in an 18-year-old. Being accused of infanticide immediately after having given birth, there was an investigation running against an 18-year-old unmarried high school girl who was socially adapted and well integrated into a family of five persons, i.e., living at home and on her way to graduation. Without anyone's help she had born a child in breech presentation and had, half an hour after birth, wrapped the baby, which showed all signs of maturity, in cloths and placed it at night in cold weather at the front door of a welfare centre. She rang the doorbell and after the light had gone on believed it would be found there. However, the baby died of hypothermia.

The exploration revealed no mental or psychosexual abnormalities. At the age of 17 she had had her first coital relationship to a 19-year-old; in spite of the use of condoms she became pregnant. Concerning the process of pregnancy in retrospect she reported never to have had any signs of pregnancy, no nausea, no vomiting, especially no increase of abdominal measurement and certainly no child movement, on the contrary: Until the end she had had menstruation bleedings, regular as always, perhaps not as strong. In the 27th–30th week of pregnancy she went for a trip to the Mediterranean Sea with her schoolmates and bathed there in the nude, just like everyone else. Never did she ever think of being pregnant, nor did others suggest this possibility to her. Until 2 days prior to birth she regularly participated in school lessons including sports. On the night of the birth, she went to bed, as she told her mother "with an upset stomach". Around midnight she felt "a rumble in her stomach", felt blood between her legs, groped the scrotum and buttock of the child and then realized that she was giving birth.

The only conclusion to be drawn from this detailed objective reconstruction of pregnancy and birth (with the help of her family) was, that an intelligent, age-appropriately developed and educated about the facts of life, well-informed about possibilities and use of contraception options, 18-year-old girl with average results at high school and from an orderly social background did not perceive her pregnancy and was utterly surprised by the event of the birth.

Nevertheless, this young woman showed a destabilization of her female identity by the loss of her boyfriend (father of the child), which followed up the loss of her father, whom she had loved dearly (he died of cancer when she herself was aged 6). It is interesting to note that, already as a small child, she had developed "denial" as a defense mechanism with remarkable intensity: She was in denial about the death of her father and at school talked about alleged holiday trips with him.

The young woman rejected the offered psychotherapy, because she did not see the necessity. Therefore, a therapeutic reprocessing of the suspected background problems was not possible. Unfortunately, her further development shows in a sad way, how conflict-laden occupancy of the reproductive area of sexuality can turn out to be: One year after the tragic death of the first child, she again does not perceive the first 7 months of a further pregnancy, keeps the last weeks secret and on the occasion of her expulsion contractions informs her mother, who was present by coincidence ("listen, I'm having a baby").

In spite of immediate emergency call for medical help, it turned out to be a home childbirth assisted by the grandmother, who is still taking care of her grandchild today.

Only certain conditions due to particular constellations in this case prevented forensic consequences. The psychopathological dimension of the incident corresponds exactly to the process of the first pregnancy.

In the light of cases similar to this and other comparable ones, the hypothesis has been made that a gender-typical intrapsychic modus of conflict processing exists: While in males the matter is located more in the dimension of desire (and linked to the outer genitals), in females it is located in the dimension of reproduction (and is linked to the inner genitals). It was suggested, analogically to the term *"perversion"*, to use a new term *"reproversion"* (see Beier 1994, 2007).

Moreover, disorders of sexual reproduction are generally very often linked to disorders of sexual relationship (see Chap. 4.2.4), which can open up useful aspects for therapeutic procedures (see Chap. 6.3).

The example of the involuntary childlessness shows clearly how the reproductive dimension can become the most important dimension of sexuality, disregarding the attachment dimension and the dimension of desire: The spontaneity of passionate sexual encounters is replaced by carefully planned "acts of fertilization" timed by the calendar. The erotic, personal bonding and attraction falls back behind acts of necessity and passion is lost—not only at the time of the expected ovulation, but also before and afterward. In terms of assisted reproduction, the probability of recurring disappointment despite a great deal of energy input, the possible health risks and not least the impersonal method of planned reproduction cast a shadow over sexuality and partnership, unless there is conscious countersteering. Sexological counseling would be needed to find the balance between the three dimensions (attachment, desire, and reproduction), to make an issue of the couple's sexuality (question of meaning, function disorders), to help analyze the motivation behind the wish to have children and to point out that parenting is based on partnership, setting priorities according to these factors.

Chapter 5
Principles of Diagnostics in Sexual Medicine

In order to tackle the problem of a disturbed partnership and/or sexual life, it is essential to address the issue adequately and to explore sexual disorders, the level of syndyastic function (i.e. the extent of fulfilment of psychosocial fundamental needs for acceptance and appreciation within the relationship), as well as to evaluate physical findings and laboratory parameters in a qualified way.

At this point, the previous strict approach "first diagnosis, then therapy" should be changed into a dynamic, process orientated "diagnostic therapeutic circle" (Wesiack 1984): Every interview for assessment, empathically carried out, has a therapeutic effect in itself and every further therapeutic step produces new diagnostic material for the duration of the relationship between therapist and patient(s).

This calls for attentiveness on the part of the therapist on three information levels simultaneously: (1) on the level of given facts listening carefully, (2) on the level of the significance these facts have for the patient(s) sympathetic understanding, (3) on the level of partnership dynamics by observation of couple interaction, revealing valuable scenic information. This demands complete awareness, never to be confused with not maintaining a professional distance to the involved couple.

At the same time the therapist offers a role-model by speaking openly about sexuality as a basic element of human life. This is one of the most important foundations of sexological skills and definitely shows therapeutic effects. It has been long proven that patients actually wait for certain signals from the therapist concerning mentioning the issue of sexuality (Vincent 1964; Buddeberg 1996; Zettl and Hartlapp 1997; Fröhlich 1998). For instance, on prescribing a new medication, the therapist can provide a signal in terms of a question like: "Should the illness or its treatment lead to problems or changes in your sexual life, then we can talk about that and look for solutions".

It is essential, however, that the therapist should never retreat into the role of "the expert". He/she will always be confronted by subjective interpretations—the patient's as well as his/her own—making personal compassion inevitable.

K. M. Beier, K. K. Loewit, *Sexual Medicine in Clinical Practice*,
DOI 10.1007/978-1-4614-4421-3_5, © Springer Science+Business Media, LLC 2013

5.1   Exploration of Sexual Disorders

Successfully carrying out treatment with decisiveness is based on extensive information on the specific sexual experience and behavior of a patient/couple. In the case of partnership involvement, the information has to provide the investigator with insight into the level of sexual functions and the sexual preference structure of *both* partners; otherwise therapeutic steps remain ineffective or can even cause harm (e.g. if a preference disorder remains undetected as a reason for a dysfunction).

When couples are concerned, it must be decided whether the sexual assessment should be taken on with each partner alone or immediately with both partners together from the beginning.

Single anamnesis has the advantage that the partner may be more uninhibited and speak more openly than in the presence of the other, particularly on subjects like masturbation fantasies or topics like paraphilic inclinations and past relationships. This can, however, turn the therapist into a "keeper of secrets" which could make future work with the couple difficult.

It is not crucial for the therapist to know every detail about each partner. In fact, it is more important to gather information of relevance for both partners as a couple because it can be referred to later on during couple therapy.

In view of this, the sexological assessment as a direct *couple-interview* has great advantages, because all information issues are gathered together and processed from the beginning, which can demonstrate and increase the extent of openness and trust among the partners involved.

It is crucial to know which kind of disorder (e.g. direct or indirect disorder of sexual function; disorder of sexual partnership) is being dealt with and under which circumstances or conditions it arises (e.g. lifelong or aquired type; generalized or situational type). What is the partner's opinion on this disorder? What attitude does each partner have toward sexuality, irrespective of the disorder in question? What kind of sex education are opinions based on? Does each partner know the opinions of the other and can they talk about them? Such generalized questions are imperative in order to put specific questions into the greater context of the partnership and to be able to judge their significance for each partner, e.g.: Who takes the initiative in sexual contact? Are there differences and where and how are they expressed? Which preferences or aversions are there and how are they dealt with?

This inevitably leads to analysis of possibly existing peculiarities of sexual preference structure, which should and can quite naturally be systematically explored. (see overview).

Overview   Sexual Preference Structure: Exploration Tools

Three Axes
The human sexual preference structure is generally configured on three axes, i.e.

- **Gender** (of the desirable partner): the other or the same gender (or both);
- **Age** (of the desirable partner): children, adolescents, adults or the elderly; and
- **Way** (of the desirable partner or object or of an interaction): type, object, mode, procedure etc.,

all intermingling with one another and of which all (from nonconform to paraphilic) should be explored.

Three Levels
Sexual experience and behavior should be investigated into on three different levels, i.e.:

- The **sexual self-concept**
- The **sexual phantasies** and
- The concrete **sexual behavior.**

All intermingling with one another and of which all should be explored.

Three Forms
The concrete sexual behavior should again be explored within three forms:

- **Masturbation:** self-stimulation and self-satisfaction;
- **Extragenital sexual interaction:** e.g. stroking, cuddling, kissing and
- **Genital stimulation:** manual, oral or other stimulation, e.g. petting incl. sexual intercourse penis or penis surrogate penetrating vagina or anus,

and these should also all be explored.

The patients sense the embarrassment of the therapist more than he thinks. In fact, the extent of naturalness conveyed by the therapist during exploration has direct influence on the information flow. Alone by this, it obtains diagnostic-therapeutic relevance and underlines the necessity of acquiring a professional repertoire of knowledge and skills which can be learnt in the context of sexological advanced training (see Chap. 6.7).

It must also be said that effects on sexuality and partnership caused by aging or illnesses and/or their treatment(s) only become evident through outright questioning. Involvement of the partner in the interview comes about automatically, because sexuality is a subject concerning both partners and in situations of intimacy, wishes and expectations of the partner have to be taken into account if the partnership is to be successful.

Therefore, from a sexological angle, the following questions are diagnostically of particular interest: What is communication like within the partnership in general and in sexual matters in particular? Can personal feelings, needs and wishes be communicated and does this happen? Are boundaries respected? Are there self-strengthening mechanisms, "vicious circles" or self-fulfilling prophecies and how do these affect partnership communication? Can misunderstandings due to misinterpretations of partner-behavior play any part?

5.2   Exploration of the Three Dimensions of Sexuality

Diagnostically and therapeutically it is essential to determine the patient's/couple's subjective classification concerning the three dimensions (reproduction, desire and attachment) of sexuality. What kind of fantasies does each partner have compared to the light of reality and is there potential of conflict in that at all?

This approach usually involves first-time analysis and discussions about their own sexuality and partnership which may already have therapeutic effects. In the end, the aim is to gain an idea of what "sexuality" actually means to the patient/couple ("What does sleeping with your partner mean to you?"). In many patients, this may lead to the observation that some things are not so taken for granted as they might have thought to be ("we/I have never thought about that" is a frequent answer to the above question).

5.2.1   Dimension of Attachment

Is there a connection between sexuality and partnership and how is it seen? Which contents and values are indispensable within the relationship? How well are fundamental needs fulfilled on the basis of this relationship? To what extent is sexuality understood as a way of communicating these elementary needs on one hand and satisfying them by communication on the other, so that showing affection, cuddling up or having sexual intercourse can be experienced as "mimic and gesture" in this relationship? For example, is *physical* closeness and acceptance obtained during sexual interaction also an expression and implementation of *psychosocial* closeness and acceptance existing in the partnership? Is the couple conscious of this communicative new angle, is it implicitly lived in every-day life or does it fail to play any part, neither in thoughts nor in practice?

5.2.2   Dimension of Reproduction

What significance does reproductive capability have; what role do children (does the child) play within the relationship? Do the partners have different views and attitudes on this? Are there any problems, which may, for instance, cause an exaggerated desire to have children? Is there an issue of involuntary childlessness? Does this affect the balance between the dimension of reproduction and the other dimensions? Or is this even a cause for an overweight on the side of the reproductive dimension? How is contraception dealt with and how does the method of contraception affect sexuality within the relationship?

5.2.3   Dimension of Desire

What personal feelings are connected to the expression "sexual desire"? Are these feelings mainly positive, ambivalent or negative ones, are they activating or inhibiting and in which context do these arise. Are both partners able to let go and give in to their feelings without fearing loss of control? How much significance, which priority and what position within the three dimensions is given to genital sex? Has the degree of significance concerning desire changed during the course of the relationship and how exactly? Are there disturbing discrepancies between the partners? Are the partners aware of the complexity of experiencing lust? Do both of the couple have definite ideas and, most of all, experience on the issue of "desire for attachment"?

5.2.4   Individual and Partner-Related Interaction of the Three Dimensions of Sexuality

Are there imbalances detectable in the individual partner or within the couple that could be connected to a current sexual disorder? Here, the possibility of (a) the discrepancy between fantasized and in reality experienced sexuality and (b) the predominance of one of the dimensions at the expense of the other or (c) a completely different distribution concerning the couple must be taken into consideration (see Case Report in Chap. 6.5)

5.3   History of Diseases and Somatic Findings

All significant diseases treated medically at the present time or previously should be taken into account, but particularly those, which might be connected with the sexual disorder. This includes all urological, gynecological or psychosomatic illnesses and surgery as well as any medication and/or substance abuse or addiction. It is also important to record all information concerning pregnancies (abortions and miscarriages) and childbirth.

In addition any therapy relevant to sexual disorders and previous psychotherapeutic treatment need to be looked into.

Biopsychosocial anamnesis needs to include diagnostics for somatic findings. This concerns *sexual functions* as well as *general physical functions*. An overview on the necessary physical diagnostics concerning sexual dysfunctions in males is shown in Table 5.1 (Rösing et al. 2009).

Table 5.1 Organ diagnostics in sexual dysfunction in men. (Rösing et al. 2009)

Physical diagnostics	Diagnostic method	For exclusion	Indication
Clinical examination	Inspection, palpation, pulse, exercise tolerance test	Urogenital, neurological and cardiovascular diseases	General examination in connection with risk factors (e.g. age, overweight)
Laboratory	Blood sugar	Diabetes mellitus	General examination
	Lipids	Dyslipidosis	General examination
	Testosterone	Hypogonadism	If necessary in arousal disorder or ED, depending on further hypogonadism symptoms
	Prolactin	Prolactinoma	
Imaging	Duplex sonography with intracavernous pharmacotesting	Cavernous insufficiency	If necessary in ED; in the case of no response to oral medication and wish for SKAT
	Neurophysiology (e.g. corpus-cavernosum-EMG)	Neurogenic deficit (e.g. following an accident)	If necessary in ED when expertise or scientific issues are concerned
	Penile angiography	Pelvic vascular occlusion	Only in planned revascularisation surgery

ED erectile dyfunction

5.4 Special Circumstances

Sometimes in sexual medicine there are patients to be dealt with who have no partner, which may have different reasons:

1. *The patient has not found a partner yet*: This evokes the question concerning relationship capabilities, ego strength, self-esteem etc. Depending on the competence of the therapist, it might be possible to work on their ego boosting and contact capability, meaning of sexuality etc. or to refer them to a more suitable psychotherapy. In cases like this, it is not a sexological indication in a strict sense, even when sexual problems are cause for complaint (such as masturbation difficulties, erectile disorder, premature orgasm), but rather an indirect indication particularly with regard to a (usually aspired) future relationship.
2. *The patient has lost his/her partner or has no partner because of function disorder(s)*: This may be attributed to a personal background issue, which possibly might also have to be tackled by a trained psychotherapist (as in 1.). It is diagnostically instructive to look into relevant experiences, anxieties etc. concerning previous partnerships. Possibly the patient wrongly considers the sexual dysfunction as the reason for loosing his/her partner, the true reason, however, is due to problems on the level of relationship. In sexual medicine intervention tools for

the treatment of sexual function disorders are very restricted when dealing with one single person. In any case, "masturbation training" should not be labeled "self-gratification"; it should be regarded as a "preparation for partnership" and discovering self, own well-being and taking responsibility for one's own sexual pleasure rather than putting it on the partner. Nevertheless, the situation with a partner would again be different.

3. *Sometimes, the partners of a patient might not want to come along*: In this case, the following questions have to be answered: Is it a matter of the way the request was put?

   – Does the patient, does the therapist really want to have him/her there?
   – Does the therapist believe that the partner will come?
   – Try again, perhaps acting the invitation request through in a short role-play.

4. *The partner definitely does refuse to come along*: There is no sexologically relevant therapeutic help available in that case until the situation changes and the patient should know that he/she can come back with his/her partner at any time, if it does.

Case Report 11

After failure of his first marriage, the 45-year-old pharmacist had married his apprentice, who, 20 years younger, "challenges him sexually too much". If it were up to her, she would want to have vaginal sexual intercourse at least once if not twice a day. This is also his favoured method (according to the exploration of his sexual preference structure), but not in such frequency. As a result, it has come to erectile disorder ("in fact, I really don't want to do it then") registered reproachfully by his wife and nourishing her jealousy, that he might have a girlfriend somewhere, for whom he "really has no capacity" left over.

He is already regularly taking PDE5 inhibitors to improve the erectile function, he had not seen an urologist about this, after all, he is "at the source" (in a pharmacy).

The interview with the wife was marked by lacking readiness on her part to cooperate. She remarked that "daily sexual intercourse" surely goes with marriage, without being able to explain, what it meant to her. She sees it the other way around: She would not feel loved, if it did not come to sexual intercourse, which is why she sees to it that it happens regularly. Erection restrictions are, from her point of view, also an obvious sign of lacking affection, otherwise "it would work". There was no wish to have children and the sexual interactions she had initiated had by no means always led to sexual arousal climaxes, these being not so significant, as long as vaginal penetration came about.

During a session with the couple, only the husband was able to report, that the young woman had been brought up under difficult primary familial conditions and had never received enough love and affection. In her mind coital intimacy and devotion are on the same level and she feels abandoned when it does not take place.

In practice it is very often the case that a patient suffering from erectile disorder "just needs a prescription for Viagra". In the interest of the patient it is necessary to ask: What are his reasons? What about anxieties? What about communication between the partners and is there a basis of trust? Does his partner know about the desired medication and what is her attitude or why should she not know about it? Is he perhaps misjudging his partner's reaction? Being able to have an erection—what significance does that have for him? The therapist will try to make a point of talking to both partners and a prescription should depend on a joint session. In any case it should be aimed at making a point of how important trust and openness within the partnership is in order to tackle more hidden difficulties. What about trust and openness in the relationship between the therapist and the patient (a mirror of own personal relationships)? Possibly there is a chance of involving the partner in the second step (how did it work at home?) (For more details see Chap. 6.3).

5.5   Sexological Expert Assessments

Requests for sexological expert assessments are dependant on different legal procedures in each country and usually placed by courts, some by investigation authorities (prosecution) or government authorities (education board, church institutions etc). In quantity, the majority concern assessments with queries on criminal responsibility and prognosis. Here, minimum requirements are to be observed in order to adequately take a stand on subjects questioned by the court such as to the existence of any criminal responsibility-diminishing or even suspending pathological disorders in the offender or any restrictions of judiciousness and accountability caused by this condition at the time of the offence (see Boetticher et al. 2005), as well as being able to take position on the issue of prognosis (see Boetticher et al. 2006). When sexual offenders are concerned, the diagnosis specially focuses on the existence of any paraphilia (such as pedophilia), perhaps being covered up by the assessed person, so that self-disclosure of confidential information should be cautiously evaluated, which makes the involvement of previous or current sexual partners particularly relevant (as is designated in the minimum requirements mentioned above) and causes consequences for prognosis as well as therapy (see Chap. 5.5.1).

Always increasing are issues within lawsuits of Family Courts, as, for example, in the case of visitation arrangements, child custody or resident permits whenever the father is alleged to have pedophilic inclinations. With the well-being of the child in mind, the mother might presume an offence risk, which may be the basis for prohibiting unaccompanied contact to the child, (not to mention custody rights for the father).

Requests for sexological expert assessment in such matters usually concern the question, whether or not a pedophile inclination is detectable and whether or not this would endanger this father's child/children. Sexological expertise is all the more called for, because other sexual preference disorders (e.g. fetishism, see Chap 4.4) can be the subject of a lawsuit in Family Court whenever a child's mother makes allegations (as mentioned above) concerning the risk for the child/children in contact situations with the child's/children's father. It is always taken for granted that a father with a possible sexual preference disorder has no behaviour control and would, whenever given the chance, act out his sexual impulses (e.g. even fetishistic preferences) without scruples about involving his own children. It has to be anticipated that queries on such topics within civil lawsuits will increase and that qualified sexological expert assessors will be called for.

Rather seldom, but also relevant in sexual medicine, are expert assessments concerning care laws, e.g. in queries about sterilization of mentally retarded persons, where not only a specific pregnancy risk has to be dealt with, but also an opinion might have to be given concerning the sexological options in involuntary pregnancy.

A large number of assessment requests concern transsexuality (see Chap. 5.5.2), especially in countries with specific transsexual laws. These are commissioned by the District Courts in charge of personal status affairs and are a great challenge to sexual medicine, after all, opinion has to be given on matters such as irreversible gender identity disorders, because these requirements are legally essential for a change of Christian name. Furthermore insurance companies require these assessments for their decisions concerning coverage of costs involved in the process of surgical body changing measures.

It should be general knowledge that merely the statement of an individual that he/she believes to be transsexual ("in the wrong physical gender"), is by far not enough basis for a secure diagnosis, which, in itself, describes the basic problem when dealing with these cases: The individuals concerned often feel themselves being wrongfully "put to the test", because they themselves are convinced that their problem is explainable by an (alleged) transsexuality and they are hardly ever prepared to even take alternative diagnosis into consideration, which is something clinicians are supposed to do. It is all the more necessary to comply with the given standards (see Chap. 4.3), because doing this and gaining the greatest possible certainty in the sense of the patient(s) long-termed well-being may be more effort, but definitely justified in comparison to a hastily given diagnosis of transsexuality, which later exposes itself as being wrong, i.e. misdiagnosis of serious consequences.

5.5.1 Expert Assessments in Accordance with Penal Law

Independent from any specific state's penal law, it is of essential significance to find out, whether the offence was based on a sexual preference disorder in the offender (e.g. pedophilia or sadism, see Chap. 4.4) or whether it was "substitute conduct" in the offender, which, again, could be caused by various reasons (e.g. personality disorder, sociosexual inexperience, mental retardation etc., see Chap. 4.5). Following aspects should therefore be observed:

a. Detailed analysis of file references concerning the circumstances of the crime, crime scene situation, statements and conduct of the offender. The offence may be the first (acted out) manifestation of a paraphilia, which makes this significant for evaluation.

b. Extensive sexological anamnesis with particular focus on following issues: General circumstances and development of sexual socialization within the family; development of gender identity and sexual orientation; points in time and process as well as personal experience of physical sexual development (including any disorders and diseases), particularly in puberty; development and content of erotic-sexual fantasies (take-up, frequency), mode of masturbation during childhood, adolescence, adulthood as well as current masturbation habit (including the accompanying fantasies); data, staging, initiative and experiencing sociosexual development ("playing doctors", first crush, first date, first kiss, petting, sexual intercourse, allocating the gender of the partner); experience of sexual or other forms of assault during childhood, youth and adulthood (as witness, victim or offender); extensive (sexual) anamnesis concerning delinquency: In such cases other expert assessments and previous criminal sentences need to be taken into consideration. In Germany, the external expert can use information from previous law suits against the defendant which are otherwise subject to legal exclusion of evidence. The exploration should be extended to legally unknown offences—having given the defendant appropriate legal instruction; previous treatment of psychiatric and or sexual disorders or diseases; consumption of pornography; contact to prostitutes; partnership anamnesis including sexual functions (begin, initiative, duration, staging and experiencing of partnership(s), objectifiable data concerning partnership anamnesis such as engagements, marriages, parenthood etc.; sexual practices, disorders of sexual functions, possible external relationships, violence within partnerships).

As a rule, questioning of current and/or previous sexual partners to support diagnostic security (and also for the exclusion of paraphilic inclination) is called for (third-party assessment), because to date there are no scientifically objectifiable methods for ascertainment or exclusion of a (denied or wrongly claimed) paraphilia. During assessment the right of relatives to refuse to give evidence and the investigation prohibition for the assessor need to be observed. Any ambiguities in the completed assessment have to be made transparent and explained in detail to the court.

After a paraphilia is diagnosed it has to be determined, whether it is in accordance with the criteria of diminished accountability, differing according to each state's penal system. In German law, for example, paraphilias are subdivided as "severe psychic abnormalities". Ultimately, it has to be looked into, whether or not and how this paraphilia had influence on the accountability *at the time of the offence (!)* The expert witness merely gives the court scientifically established recommendations and states requirements for legal adjudication of diminished or annulled accountability, professional criteria and own limits of findings and empathy capabilities are to be discussed and put to the court as an expert recommendation aimed at decision-making procedure. According to the minimum requirements for criminal accountability assessments (see Boetticher et al. 2005) expert classification of a paraphilia needs to investigate:

- The proportion of paraphilia within the sexual preference structure (e.g. exclusive type vs. the non-exclusive type of pedophilia according to DSM IV-TR);

- The intensity of the paraphilic pattern experienced by the individual (light to strongly compulsive);
- The integration of the paraphilia into the general self-concept (ego-syntone vs. ego-dystone);
- The handling of the issue of paraphilia in the individual concerned—also within the context of a law suit, an expert assessment or a previous treatment (i.e. previous to the current assessment caused by the index offence);
- The previous capability of the defendant to control paraphilic impulses (i.e. previous to the current assessment caused by the index offence).

A "severe psychic abnormalitiy" can be taken into consideration in following findings:

- The sexual preference structure is to a great extent determined by the paraphilic impulses;
- An ego-dystone processing leads to blocking out the paraphilia for oneself, thus being withdrawn from deliberate control;
- A progredient increase and inundation by compulsive paraphilic impulses followed by lacking satisfaction causes *acting out the impulse* on the behavioural level;
- Other kinds of sociosexual rewards are not available to the individual concerned (significant and verifiable lack of sociosexual alternatives) —also due to personality factors and/or sexual function disorder(s).

The appraisal of accountability requires a detailed analysis of the factual circumstances of the offence (meeting and relationship between offender and victim) as well as procedure and location of the offence (behaviour prior to, during and after the offence, modus operandi, i.e. among other things considering verbal utterances by the offender, evidence of ritualized conduct, taking or leaving behind of certain objects, use of violence and, if occurred, injury patterns etc.). Coding a paraphilia as a "severe psychic abnormality" does not automatically lead to a severe diminishment of direction capability at the time of the offence. Nevertheless, under certain circumstances, the degree of severity of a paraphilia (e.g. a pedophilia) can be extrapolated by the offender's behavior during the offence. Opportunistic surrogate conduct or forced sensuous, possibly even orgastic "kick" conduct, hedonistic need for pleasure, in otherwise normal sexuality and relationship (derived from third party assessment) do not indicate diminishment of accountability. Reckless, situationally incomprehensible, irrational offence behavior alone is no criteria for admission into the domain of nonconformity or paraphilia. Later made statements of the defendant concerning his motives and intentions at the time of the offence with—in some cases—bizarre reinterpretations or re-attributions (e.g. regarding alleged own initiative of the victim or missing sexual reference to the offence) alone do not justify assumption of a severely diminished direction capability at the time of the offence and can be—perhaps by decree of a command of silence or other possibilities—exposed. If in the defendant there had been a forensic assessment made for a previous trial connected to the current matter, in the course of which his paraphilic inclination had been made clear to him and/or if this inclination had been cause for therapeutic intervention in his past history, then, normally (at least in averagely intelligent individuals) it is *not* appropriate to assume a blocked out coping strategy with relevant effects on the accountability at the time of the offence. In chronic-deficit performance due to sexual function disorder(s) with impending loss of partner, particularly in cases of the ego-dystone pedophilic non-exclusive type in crises or strong temptation situations, a diminished accountability could seriously be taken into consideration.

A forensically relevant impairment of accountability can be taken into consideration when following aspects apply (see Boetticher et al. 2005):

- In worsening conflict dynamics and emotional instability during the time prior to the offence along with already existing sexual frustration caused by the impossibility of sociosexual realization (e.g. pedophilic exclusive type, obsessing fetishism or sadism);
- Offence procedure even in socially strongly controlled situations;
- Abrupt, impulsive offence procedures (the execution of the offence as a paraphilic scenario, obviously "thought through" beforehand—like in fantasy—is not necessarily an exclusion criterion for diminished accountability);
- Archaic-destructive procedure with seemingly ritualized offence execution and evidence for the blocking out of external stimuli.

Relevant constellational factors (e.g. alcohol intoxication) are to be taken into consideration as much as the existence of striking personality features or evidence of personality disorder or restricted intelligence, which, cumulated, could cause an extensive diminishment of accountability at the time of the offence.

5.5.2 Assessments According to Legal Aspects of Transsexuality

Internationally many different legal systems deal with gender correction issues in connection with transsexuality (some countries, however, have no legal regulations at all).

In Germany, since 1981, there is a law on changes of first given name and the statement of the gender under certain circumstances (so-called "Law on Transsexuality"). This law was issued exclusively for mitigation of suffering in a certain patient population—individuals with transsexual gender identity disorder.

It allows for two options:

1. The changing of the first given name according to the personally perceived belonging to the other gender—with no change of the birth gender in the official birth register and according documents of the civil registry office.
2. Additionally the changing of civil status, meaning the change of the registered gender in the birth registry documents.

The court is only allowed to comply with an application, after having obtained expert witness assessments from two experts, who are—due to their education and professional experience—sufficiently familiar with the particular problems of transsexuality. These experts need to work independently from one another on the case; in their assessment it is necessary to have adequately looked into the subject of whether—according to justified findings in medical science—the perception of belonging to the opposite gender will, with greatest likelihood, never change again.

Subsequently, a great responsibility is imposed upon the expert witnesses: After all, they not only have to deal with a condition and its history, but are called upon to determine its future (lifelong) irreversibility, and that with prognostic likelihood. According to the German Sexological Societies' "Standards of Treatment and Expert Assessment of Transsexuals" (Becker et al. 1997) the following minimum requirements need to be noted:

The purpose of the expert assessment is to portray the development of the gender identity and its disorder (taking into consideration the particularities of male-to-female and female-to-male transsexuals) in the context of the existing psychosocial environment covering all influence factors within the successive life phases.

The expert witness should, if necessary, procure additional information, in which statements by important close or related persons (third party assessment) and psychological-medical findings may play an important role. The evaluation should be scientifically founded and include a critical discussion. A summary on the individual concerned or a patient's report on subjective perception or a reproduction of the self-interpretation of the personal curriculum vitae alone is not a legitimate judgement of expert witness. Equally important as the empathy into the subjectivity of the transsexual conviction is the critical attention concerning objectifiable aspects of behaviour. The existence of these requirements necessary for changing the first given name should become obvious in the appraisal (Becker et al. 1997).

In the context of the expert appraisal it is necessary to rule out by differential diagnostics:

- Any unease, difficulties or non-conformity with common expectations concerning gender roles.
- Partial or passing disorder of gender identity (such as in crises of adolescence).
- Difficulties with gender identity resulting from denial of a homosexual orientation.
- Psychotically influenced misapprehension of the gender identity as well as grave personality disorders with consequences concerning gender identity.
- Transvestitism and transvestic fetishism as well as autogynephilia.

The course of the "real-life experience" is essential for the diagnostics: The patient lives continually and in all social settings in the desired gender, in order to gather necessary experiences and to evaluate these with the therapist.

When a diagnosis has been secured by this method and a transsexual identity disorder thus established, sex reassignment therapy achieves a convergence to the physical appearance of the other gender. This includes hormone replacement therapy and specific surgery (see Chap. 4.3).

Generally, in biological males with transsexual identity disorder gynecomastia (often sufficiently obtained by hormone treatment) as well as penectomy and orchidectomy and the shaping of a neo vagina are called for. In biological females with transsexual identity disorder the removal of the breasts will most likely be called for, as well as the extirpation of the uterus and the ovaries, while external genital surgical procedures may include scrotoplasty, urethroplasty, placement of testicular prostheses, and phalloplasty (WPATH 2011).

Chapter 6
Principles of Therapy in Sexual Medicine

6.1 Basic Approach

Generally, similar to every medical branch, sexual medicine can be interpreted and practiced in two ways: focusing on disease or focusing on the patient, in sexual medicine ideally: "focusing on the couple and their partnership".

6.1.1 Disease-Centred Aspects of Sexual Therapy

The first-mentioned approach deals primarily with "disorders" of sexual function, of gender identity, of sexual preferences and of sexual behaviour. The pathogenesis is primarily in the centre of scientific interest. Anatomy, physiology, neuro-endocrinology etc. are favoured subjects. Diagnostics are made according to common classifications by assessment of facts, clinical examinations, laboratory results including hormone analysis, function tests etc. and are recorded in a "case history". The therapy is aimed at fast and efficient elimination of the disorder, i.e. at the re-establishment of normal function. Till the end of the sessions with the therapist, pharmacological, surgical and technical methods are available and most times applied to the one single person with such symptoms. Examples for this are, for instance concerning the most frequent indications, the disorders of sexual function, the reflex-like prescription of PDE5-inhibitors in erectile disorder without carrying out any differentiated assessment, not to speak of talks to the couple involved; or the treatment of vaginism with dilating measures, without ever having spoken to the male partner; or the administration of hormones, e.g. testosterones for hypoactive sexual desire disorder as first choice therapy—the list could go on and on.

6.1.2 Patient-Centred Aspects of Sexual Therapy

In the second approach of applied sexual medicine using an integral medical approach, the patient, i.e. *the couple and their partnership* becomes the main focus:

K. M. Beier, K. K. Loewit, *Sexual Medicine in Clinical Practice,*
DOI 10.1007/978-1-4614-4421-3_6, © Springer Science+Business Media, LLC 2013

No abstract disease or disorder is to be treated, and not just one suffering individual in his/her uniqueness, it is more about understanding a disorder which has developed within a partnership or a particular relationship constellation and therefore is always affecting two individuals and their relationship to one another. In other words, not only the individual with the symptoms, but *both partners* are involved: Two distinctive persons with their specific gender-typical biographies and their resulting (also sexual) "worldviews" are interacting, during which physical, psychological and social factors mutually influence each other, both in the individual and in the couple (enabled, e.g. by the function of the mirror neurons).

Thinking and acting in sexual medicine have to be based on the reality of this given complexity, even if it can only be indicated here. An evaluation of any given situation is therefore only possible, when the couple is viewed during interaction. In this case, the salutogenesis and not the pathogenesis is the centre of interest, i.e. not rectification of a malfunction but supporting healing and health-maintaining elements, leading to partnership contentment in general.

This does not at all mean neglecting any likely causes involved, but to complete them by the somatic findings.

This can be illustrated quite well by using the example of low sexual desire after giving birth and during breastfeeding: The whole physical, in particular the hormonal (high progesterone and prolactin level) conversion is causally involved in the reduction of sexual desire, but no less does the stress (eustress or distress) emerge from the whole current life situation.

Was pregnancy the result of a joint wish for reproduction or was it something that happened against her own will? Did an abortion come into consideration at any time? Who responded how to this? How did the partner and "the family" react to the announcement of gravidity (high personal offence potential at ambivalent or disapproving reaction) and how actively did the pregnant woman feel to be supported by him/her? How did she (and her partner!) cope with the changes of the body scheme and her self-image (her role as a partner, a lover and/or a mother), etc.?

Surveys have shown that in this critical life phase physical affection often decreases and communication can deteriorate, in primiparae more strongly than in multiparae (Seiwald 1996).

There are still other factors that need to be taken into consideration: A hostile attitude towards children in society and possibly lacking appreciation and support by the environment as well as the significance of other likely stress factors, such as issues concerning health, vocational aspects, finances and living conditions, etc. It would be much too short sighted, to just concentrate on "hormones", which do, of course, also need to be taken into consideration.

Instead of the common "clinical diagnosis" there is an "overall diagnosis" dynamically developing itself, in which not only facts, but on top of that their subjective significance, that means the "whole (hi)story of significance or suffering" are important.

Balint (1957) calls them the "standard" and the "comprehensive" diagnosis.

It compiles the status of the current information about this couple and their partnership or about this singular patient, i.e. it also includes the clinical diagnosis, but is not limited to that.

Obviously the right approach is not a matter of being *either disease-centred or patient-centred*, it is about *avoiding one-sidedness* in both directions: neither a pure somatotherapeutic nor a pure psychotherapeutic course do justice to life's realities: a biopsychosocial, couple- and partnership-related approach is called for.

Taking all this into account, it can be said, that the prescription of PDE5-inhibitors can be very appropriate following a detailed talk—generally a talk with both partners—which ascertains, whether or not the partner really wants a re-establishment of erectile efficiency. Furthermore, it has to be figured out which significance do sexuality and coitus have within the relationship, what sort of sexual preference and satisfaction is there and last not least how is the physiological process of an erection influenced by medication. In that case, it will not come to misinterpretations by the partner of a man with erectile disorder such as "you need a pill to have sex with me, so you do not love me". These distorted views can only be avoided by involving the partner from the beginning.

The same is true for assessing a problem such as vaginism: How—and with which background—has the couple managed until now?, what is the significance of sexuality within the relationship for both partners?, Is it simply about the reproductive dimension of sexuality, about a desire for children (e.g. by the future grandparents)?, Did the partner have any say in solution concepts?, etc.

Particularly in cases of decreased sexual desire, firstly there is a focus on the obvious reasons within the relationship itself, for instance the personal understanding of "sex and love", and then the question of fulfilment and frustration of psychosocial fundamental needs has to be raised, before hormones are given or the prolactin level is determined. Even in obviously hormone-influenced libido changes, such as post-partal or during lactation, the impact of partnership quality is quite significant.

It is not yet well enough known that positive partnership situations and experiences of intimacy actually can release hormones, e.g. the bonding hormone oxytocin, which works as trust stimulating, anxiety and stress reducing and in interaction with dopamine, endorphins, additional neurotransmitters and sexual hormones has vitalizing and harmonizing effects.

Years ago, the psychiatrist Bauer (2005) wrote: "good interpersonal relations are the most efficient 'drug' completely lacking side-effects for dealing with psychological and physical stress."

Meanwhile, this statement has been corroborated, e.g. by a study on the "influence of a 'warm touch' support enhancement intervention" which has shown that "warm physical contact between marital partners" has enhanced salivary oxytocin, reduced alpha amylase (as an indicator of sympathetic activation) and lowered 24-hours systolic blood pressure especially in husbands. The authors conclude, that "increased support and affection among couples may confer health benefits", i.e. have an advantageous influence "on multiple stress-sensitive systems" (Holt-Lunstad et al. 2008). But also the very reverse is true: Nasally administered oxytocin was ineffective (in enhancing donating behaviour) in individuals who experienced high levels of parental

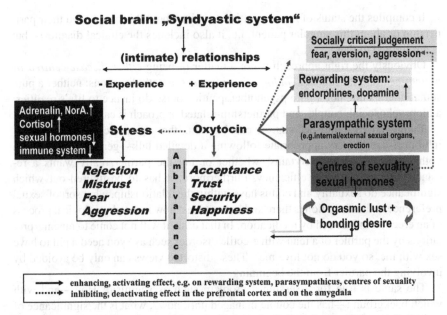

Fig. 6.1 Oxytocin qualifies as one of the neurobiological substrates in the attachment dimension of sexuality

love-withdrawal (van IJzendoorn et al. 2011) and childhood maltreatment may result in, e.g. atypical responsiveness of the hypothalamus–pituitary–adrenal-axis to stress and even in structural brain differences (McCrory et al. 2011) as risk factors for adult psychopathology.

Such studies underline once more the importance of a biopsychosocial approach: purely somatic as well as purely psychotherapeutic concepts are too narrowly considered.

This "hormone self-therapy" could and should be prescribed by each partner themselves, especially on occasions of "hormone deficiency" and child maltreatment and abuse should be prevented as well and not least for the sake of adult sexual health, keeping in mind that a history of childhood abuse could be associated with lower oxytocin concentrations in cerebrospinal fluid in affected adults (Heim et al. 2009). Figure 6.1 explains the connections between oxytocin as one of the neurobiological substrates relevant for the attachment dimension of sexuality.

Keeping this in mind, the following describes a biopsychosocial, couple- and relationship-centred sexual therapy.

6.1.3   The Dual Role of the Therapist as an Expert and an Attendant

A disease-oriented *and* patient-oriented perspective means a challenge concerning *two* emphases or roles of the physician: the medical expert and the empathic assistant.

In German-speaking countries, during standard undergraduate medical training, a certain image of a physician is conveyed, which depicts him/her as a caring helper and healer but at the same time as a person thinking in terms of "objective" natural science, occasionally a distanced expert observer and responsible problem solver and solution finder, the success of therapy depending on his/her skills and knowledge. He/she knows, what is best for his/her patients, clarifies, educates, teaches, gives authoritative orders and advice to be followed in trust by his/her patients. He/she might find it difficult to cope with "informed patients", especially when confronted with resistance and contradiction, strong emotions might make him/her insecure and helpless, i.e. they activate his/her (subconscious) defence mechanisms and this additionally puts a strain on the doctor–patient relationship as an essential healing remedy.

The second—also aspired—image of the doctor aims at exactly that patient-focused conduct as an empathic companion, a good patient listener who "reads between the lines", who tries to assess the patient—in this case the couple—in their overall situation. To achieve this he/she applies his/her own reflected experiences at each ongoing doctor–patient relationship as a diagnostic instrument, as has been previously worked out, particularly by Balint (1957, 1975). Within the "Balint Groups", named after him, these abilities can be learnt and practiced (Loewit 2005; Kress and Loewit 2012), which is done more and more in regular medical training, while in psychology and psychotherapy it is general state of the art. Sexual medicine, however, is no "psycho subject" and, sexual therapy is not a specialized form of psychotherapy, which is why specialists such as urologists, andrologists, gynecologists, dermatologists, general practitioners (GPs) and psychiatrists, etc., who want to gain additional qualification in sexual medicine to add to their specialized field, definitely need to learn and train role security in this new identity as a companion, catalyst, mirror, midwife and aide to problem-solving by the patient or the couple themselves (see Chap. 6.5).

Beyond the necessity for every physician and therapist to develop his/her "second identity", this comes especially true for the couple-centred approach in diagnosis and treatment in sexual medicine. This approach, however, plays no noteworthy role in any other medical discipline.

This is why there is no means of reassurance in unsettling situations and this may lead to wanting to return to the well-rehearsed role security of the expert and knowledgeable scientist, i.e. the responsible one for solving the problems of the couple. Fact is, concerning the particular couple in question, one is actually the "not knowledgeable one", having to rely on enquiries and observations, leaving the solving of the couple's problems to the couple itself.

> The couple heals itself, the therapist offers the necessary "sheltered workshop" and supplies the continuity of the process. He/she would be out of his/her depth with the role of the expert as far as the couple relationship goes.

It is also crucial for him/her to be conscious of both his/her roles, the one of the expert and the one of the assistant, that he/she has both available, feels comfortable in both, and is able to apply any one of both wherever needed, particularly in a couple setting.

This is a skill which needs to be taught and practiced. It represents an indispensable demand to every training programme in sexual therapy.

6.1.4 Roots of the Syndyastic Approach

A patient-centred, couple- and relation-oriented sexual medicine takes human conditions in particular under anthropological aspects into account: It has already been pointed out that man—as other species before him, in particular his mammal and primate ancestors—is created for and dependant on attachment. In this context, partnership between two individuals is of significant meaning: The story of life begins for all of us as a relationship between mother and child and in every life history there is always a yearning for especially extensive bonding, i.e. intimate friendships and love relationships, generally found in partnerships or in becoming a couple. This is archaic human knowledge. As already stated, within European culture the great philosopher and scholar Aristotle (384–322 BC) coined the word "syndyastikós" in his book *Nicomachean Ethics*, meaning "laid out for partnerships", i.e. "being disposed to live in pairs", emerging into "belonging" within a partnership.

In contemporary understanding, he would be referring to the already reiterated trans-cultural universal psychosocial fundamental needs for belonging, unconditional acceptance, esteem and development of one's personality, closeness, warmth, security and safety, which are—no matter what gender or sexual orientation—regarded as biopsychosocial existence minima. Fulfilment of these needs is the central issue concerning all interpersonal relationships, especially in friendships and romantic relationships, influencing their quality. Therefore the term "syndyastic" describes the evolutionarily developed internal programming of human beings on attachment and relationships. This programming is aimed at fulfilment of existentially compulsory biopsychosocial fundamental needs and has developed in Western culture preferably as a couple-relationship (see Beier and Loewit 2004).

The described biopsychosocial causes of sexual disorders call for an appropriate therapeutic approach, a combination of methods, of "narrative medicine" with those of somatic interventions (see Rösing et al. 2008).

Taking as an example the treatment of post-prostatectomy erectile disorder caused by prostatic cancer, a German study showed that in long-term exclusive use of medication or mechanical treatment options, the patients were clearly less satisfied than their treating urologists would have imagined (see Herkommer et al. 2006). Even concerning the selection of therapy options, the patients' comments were clearly discrepant to the judgment of their treating physicians. Questions concerning the importance of partnership, of non-genital sexuality (the exchange of affectionate words and gestures) and genital sexuality (intercourse) put to prostate cancer patients and their partners *before and after radical prostatectomy* showed that only the importance of genital sexuality decreased and not the non-genital kind. Partnership in general and the meaning of physical attachment maintained an unchanged high value (Rösing and Berberich 2004). The high rating of satisfaction of psychosocial intimacy, closeness and security in comparison to aiming at sexual erotic satisfaction has also been validated by other studies (Deneke 1999).

> Sexological interventions, therefore, are imperatively based on the consideration of biopsychosocial aspects of sexuality and on systematic involvement of partnership issues and communication (e.g. the couple is the patient). Such modifications of conventional patient concepts also lead to a different understanding of therapy.

The familiar concept of the "therapist-patient" relationship is extended—especially in the case of sexual disorders—to a new "therapist–couple" relationship. Advocacy for the patient turns into plural advocacy for the couple and their partnership, as long as this is the mandate given to the therapist. A Paracelsus (1493–1541) quotation *"The patient is the doctor and the doctor is his assistant"* reflects the real therapeutically effective work with a couple—the *"assistant"* accompanying, making suggestions, enquiring more about than settling problems, supporting, confronting, possibly acting as interpreter between different personalities and genders. He enables the couple to gain new insights and to make new experiences designed to improve life quality. So, the therapeutic aim is focused on partnership and sexuality.

This approach reveals a clear difference to the "function-centred counselling", commonly carried out in clinical work, which is reduced to communicating information and treatment options concerning sexual functions (including the prescription of PDE-5-inhibitors in erectile disorders): A sexological consultation goes further than that, because it is based on a certain concept of sexuality (see Chap. 3), which takes the dimension of attachment beyond any function disorders into account and considers this dimension as being an essential resource for sexual contentedness (see Chap. 6.2). In many cases, this turns out to be a helpful approach for the patients because an idea for behavioural change is given—within quite a short time (usually not more than 2–3 sessions)—and this is often enough to get things going. If this proves not to be sufficient, supportive sexual therapeutic interventions can be supplied systematically to achieve the aspired modification of attitude and behaviour over a longer period of time (see Chap. 6.3).

6.2 Sexological Counselling

6.2.1 Medical Indication and Key Aspects

Seeking help in times of need is generally regarded as a wise action—but not so where problems in partnership and sexuality are concerned. Obviously, it is not generally accepted for people to have difficulties in this field and if they do arise, they must be dealt with alone, it is no one else's business.

The inhibition threshold concerning sexological counselling or sexual therapy remains quite high. By the time the concerned persons have finally brought themselves to seek help, a great deal of time has been wasted, while the problems have not been solved, but have rather intensified. It is even more seldom that counselling is made use of in terms of informing oneself preventively, before grave problems arise.

Here, counselling does not mean giving or receiving advice, it means to take counsel or consult with somebody mutually, helping to acquire self-help, supporting the couple to find "their" solution and assisting them to take steps towards change.

Concerning the issue of time in sexological interventions, it has to be determined whether a sexological counselling or a short series of talking sessions, aiming at motivating the uptake of sexual therapy, i.e. the proper sexual therapy—which usually takes between 3 and 6 months with weekly sessions in "couple settings"—is appropriate.

Sexological counselling sessions have an informative–explanatory as well as an encouraging emphasis and can generally be fitted into regular office schedule, whereas sessions with a couple usually take up to 1 hour, which would need to be organized separately outside the regular office hours.

Sexual therapy requires regular (weekly) sessions with the couple, in which their experiences (including the intimate ones) made between sessions are carefully evaluated together, with particular attention to the syndyastic experience level.

There are also significant differences concerning the counsellor in question for the very first contact: The specialized counsellor for sexual therapy is consulted directly by motivated patients or couples with problems of a sexual nature, while a general practitioner or any other specialist has to take the lead and may have to refer to the issue of partnership and sexuality on his own initiative. This might quite obviously be the case in unspecific somatization, metabolic disorder, urological or gynecologist conditions, etc. but might also cause severe resistance in the patient. Many patients are fixated on diseases based on organic causes which are able to be healed by medication remedies respectively do not call for any own responsibility, this rather being passed on to the specialist at hand.

During these exploratory situations it is necessary—independent of any sexual issues—to outline a holistic understanding of individual suffering before touching on the significance of emotional and/or sexual problems relating to the initially stated symptoms.

In the course of such conversations it is often possible in a limited time period (1–3 sessions) to supply the patient(s) with information (for instance concerning the interaction of physical and psychological factors in order to achieve sexual fulfilment) and there is also the opportunity of deconstructing one-sided ideas and inhibitions as well as pointing out the mutuality of behaviour and experience of the two partners. In a nutshell, this would describe the tasks of sexological counselling (see box).

It is the aim of sexological counselling—within a limited time period and goal-oriented sessions—to make use of the patients' own resources in order to improve their sexual and/or partnership well-being and contentedness by:

- Supplying information.
- Correcting false assumptions and wrong ideas and, in some cases
- Directly offering methods of behaviour modification in order to solve sexual problems and/or to prevent sexual disorders.

Actually, sexological counselling can be helpful in the case of information deficits in all spheres of life during which biological development processes or changes are taking or have taken place (adolescence, pregnancy, birth, etc.) as well as during stages of life in which changes of family or partnership relationships have to be coped with (e.g. after child birth, in old age, etc.) A further vast field is that concerning changes in sexuality and partnership caused by diseases or their therapy, particularly in tumour patients. This means, sexological counselling can be practical in all indication fields of sexual medicine (see Chap. 4), definitely there is not always need for sexual therapy.

Case Report 12 The 25-year-old design student had just been "dumped" by his girlfriend, because she was not prepared to further tolerate his "so frequently occurring erectile difficulties". During the 1 year relationship he had, however, never felt cause for seeking professional help, although she had asked him several times to do so. Obviously, his visit to the sexological out-patient department may come too late, although he still has regular contact to his former girlfriend. However, he does not believe that he could win her back. During the consultation it was easily worked out that the patient, who was very vain about his appearance, always tried to cover up the humiliation that went along with the recurring erectile disturbances. He admitted to evading talks on the subject with his girlfriend during their relationship. It was extremely difficult for him to talk about his anxieties with her. He did understand that in a partnership the mutual bearing-up against difficulties could turn out to be partnership strengthening and that his girlfriend's esteem might even have increased rather than decreased, if he had had the courage to reveal his weaknesses and anxieties to her. Covering up obvious problems (the erectile disorder often recurred) had to be perceived by his partner as a not understandable inadequate problem-solving strategy. After approximately 1 month, the student visited the sexological out-patient department again to inform his therapist that he had opened up to his girlfriend in the recommended way and after that—several times in the meantime—they had enjoyed sexual contact without functional problems. He wanted to know, whether he could be sure of his erectile disorder never occurring again.

Sexological counselling and sexual therapy are built on the same principles; sexual therapy is merely characterized by a more detailed and more distinctly structured course of action (see box).

Sexological Interventions Treatment in sexual medicine (sexological counselling as well as sexual therapy) is a deliberate, well-planned interactional process to take influence on sexual disorders, which—by the consensus of both patient(s)/couple and therapist—actually need to be cured.

This is achieved by psychological means (communication) and, in some circumstances, somatic methods (pharmacological, surgical and physical options) directed at a mutually defined goal (e.g. improvement of partnership contentedness; minimalizing symptoms) applying teachable techniques on the basis of a biopsychosocial theory on human sexuality.

Again it is important to point out that the significance of sexological counselling in cases of sexual disorders is to be rated very highly. It is extremely effective in many cases and can always be applied, because it would never hinder further treatment, it would rather motivate to continue, if agreed upon.

Qualifications in sexological counselling are: capability of secure communication about sexual issues; a sound basic concept of sexuality; willingness to retreat from the "role of the expert" (see box).

Qualifications for Sexological Counselling

- Flexibility in speech, i.e. being able to adapt to the language of the patient(s); security about the own chosen terms of speech.
- One's own personal conviction about the great significance of sexual satisfaction for the overall state of well-being in human beings.
- Willingness not to cover up one's personal inhibitions and difficulties (retreat from the "role of the expert").
- Knowledge concerning one's own attitude on sexuality.
- Capability of conveying the dimension of attachment (as a part of sexuality) to others.

The practice of sexological counselling therefore requires a double role, i.e. the one of playing the "modification assistant" for the patient(s)/the couple and thus helping them to detect the solution of their own problem themselves and the other one of the qualified expert called for to intervene in certain situations and to pass on information. On top of that there must be the capability of capturing the spheres of change in the couple and to directly be able to improve coping facilities (see box).

Sexological Counselling: Requirements

- Self-concept of the counsellor as "modification assistant".
- Specialized knowledge for situative intervention management and information transfer.
- Understanding and communicating points where change is necessary.
- Enhancement of coping mechanisms.
- Strategy for steps towards change.

During counselling, restoring sexual and partnership contentedness is just as much a focal issue as is the recording of current sexual problems and their possible causes of origin and development. Particularly, insight into and understanding of partnership resources enable further planning of step-by-step changes, for instance by involving the partner in counselling sessions.

For patients, difficulties during sexological counselling usually arise at the early stage of trying to verbalize their problems, which is where helpful intervention is called for. The patient(s) often point(s) out fault in the partner, making him/her responsible for the problem—this situation can only be resolved by firm partiality for both partners. Otherwise, there would be no hope of leading the couple in any direction of change, because one of the two (feeling "at fault") would refuse cooperation.

In sexological counselling, patients are very often fixated on somatic origins and hope for effective medication to deal with their problems. It must also be considered, that this might be the counsellor's pre-paved orientation, bearing the danger of not doing justice to the patient/the couple after all (see box).

Obstacles in Sexological Counselling

- Pre-paved orientation.
- Avoiding certain issues.
- Misjudgement of the symptoms.
- Taking sides.
- Chronified symptoms.

It is obvious that sexological counselling concerned with more than functional disorders is a very high-quality job, demanding not only vast knowledge, but also much empathic capability and self-restraint. Again and again it is a challenge, because it is about finding a new and individual path for each individual patient/couple. Here again it is true that diagnosis and therapy in sexological practice are knitted together creating a mutual and complementing whole: Integral diagnostic assessment is already a part of therapy and each therapeutic step leads to further diagnostic insights.

So, it can be said that sexological counselling may have a "therapeutic" impact, if it were qualified, and on the other hand cause consequential damage, if not.

Here, too, the foremost principle is to make patients/couples aware of the attachment dimension of sexuality and to apply this therapeutic aspect. Many patients/couples do not realize that genital/coital sexuality is only one of the many ways of satisfying wishes within a partnership concerning needs for authenticity, appreciation, satisfaction, closeness, security, etc.

Accordingly, sexological counselling will be adapted to the specific needs of the patient/couple, in which the following priorities, alone or combined, may be of significance:

- *Passing on knowledge* (where deficits are obvious) concerning anatomical, physiological or psychological processes of sexual reaction, and, if necessary, correcting false ideas in the sense of sexual myths (e.g. masturbation causes harm) which one or both of the partners may believe in.

  It would be quite appropriate to refer to the issue of "typical" gender differences in sexual/partnership feelings and behaviour in males and females (i.e. in this particular partner, male or female), meaning to aim at understanding and realizing differences instead of finding fault in such differences.
- *Assessment of mutual hopes and expectations* concerning sexuality and partnership.
- *Teaching communicative strategies*, if general communication difficulties are a reason for the development or continuation of the disorder concerned.

When primary illnesses are involved, specific information must be obtained:

- About the length of elapsed time between surgery and resumption of sexual contact (usually after approximately 6 weeks).
- About the use of lubrication gel, if, for instance the vaginal epithelium is altered by radiological or chemotherapy or due to menopause.
- In some cases, concerning the use of auxiliaries (tools such as an erection ring, a vacuum pump, any oral or invasive medication options)—but not before dealing with discrepancies in the relationship between the partners concerning the significance of the different dimensions of sexuality.

6.2.2 The Syndyastic Focus: A Case History on Partnership Counselling

Focusing on the (re-)fulfilment of psychosocial elementary needs ("syndyastic focus") is a key element of sexological intervention and is as relevant in sexological counselling as it is in sexual therapy. It is crucial—and usually the most difficult part for beginners—to systematically keep the steady focus amongst the abundance of given information and also to keep this perspective all the way through.

The following is a case example of sexological counselling, starting out with two individual face-to-face sessions and a concluding couple session.

Case Report 13

First session with the husband

The 63-year-old man is a retired civil servant, married for 31 years, his wife is 4 years younger. He describes briefly, what leads him to the outpatient clinic: He is "impotent" and wants to know, whether, at his age, there is anything "to be done" here, considering as he has an enlarged prostate gland and has been taking "medication against high blood pressure" since his heart attack 6 years ago. Possibly it might all be connected with the medication? On the other hand, he feels it might just as well be caused by his high masturbation frequency, which—next to coital intimate contact—has been a fixed component of his sexuality throughout his whole marriage.

More detailed assessment revealed that the patient had been treated for 5 years with a beta receptor antagonist (propanolole) due to a moderate hypertonia. Exactly since 5 years he has been in early retirement and at about this time he first experienced erectile dysfunctions. These were not at all always prominent, particularly not during masturbation, which took place approx. once a week, in former times 2–3 times a week. Since 2 years, there had been no sexual contacts with his wife. It becomes obvious that the patient had withdrawn more and more, because he was sure that he was "a burden for his wife" alone for the existence of the erectile disorder. In fact, during intimate contact he would always be worried about the erection receding or he was dissatisfied, if it were "not sufficient". He could hardly imagine his wife still being interested in him, however, both were suffering from this complete standstill of mutual sexuality. The assessment of this patient gave insight on many influencing factors, all with a tendency of unfavourably effecting sexual experience and behaviour: firstly, the current condition following the heart attack with the consequence of early retirement and high blood pressure needing treatment including possible side-effects through medication; secondly, his personal image of "impotency", for him already a fact, just because he was not in all circumstances—by own arousal or wishes from his partner—capable of an erection, even though principally sexual function was still given (such as during masturbation and morning erection); finally, the comprehensible psychological dimension of his conduct (anxious self-observation of his own sexual reaction; fear of failure toward his wife). Furthermore, there was a certain worry that he may have "used up" his sexual potency by masturbating too frequently in the past, claiming 2–3 times per week to be excessive, perhaps linked with feelings of guilt toward his wife.

This patient was suffering from a condition of frustrated needs for acceptance, closeness etc. concerning the relationship to his wife and—most important!—during the initial interview this became quite obvious to himself. Because he loved his wife and wished for (re-)accomplishment of the syndyastic dimension of their sexuality it seemed reasonable to him that this might be achieved by including the wife in the assessment and the counselling, particularly as there had never been any conversation between the couple on this subject.

First session with the wife

The wife is 59 years old and until 3 years ago had worked as a clerk in a housing management company. She is of slender stature, seems fragile and lowers her eyes during conversation. She very well knows that her husband is always worrying about his "erection problems", it is depressing for her as well that there had been no intimate contact whatsoever now since 4 years (not 2 years, like the husband said). In other ways they were such a good match, had always gotten on well together and have mutually raised three fine children. Her own sexual experience is restricted to intimate contacts to her husband; she had always liked having sex. She is quite capable of orgasm and sometimes, perhaps once a month, she reaches climax by masturbation. All the more she regrets that some time ago her husband had withdrawn altogether following several coitus attempts which had failed due to his erectile disorder. She had accepted this and let him be, even though she herself would still have liked some sexual activity and actually does not really want to do without it altogether. After all, he had had a heart attack and suffers from high blood pressure, presumably his poor health has lead to physical demands he could not cope with. Even so, their mutual sexuality was never really as pleasurable as she might have wished for— her husband had always had a very early orgasm, which he resented, too (this disorder of sexual function—a premature orgasm—was not mentioned by the husband). She, on the other hand, was still very appreciative for endearments and interested in an extended fore-play. She believes he is putting himself under extreme pressure, although she does not put pressure on him because she does not expect such performance. She would be very pleased about a revival of their sexual intimacy, even if this would not lead to intercourse. She loves her husband and would very much like to be intimately and physically close to him.

Here, only by involving the wife, the different views of both partners on their mutual sexuality became clear, but also on both sides the frustrated psychosocial needs while at the same time strong wishes existed in both for syndyastic fulfilment with and by each other. All this information now makes it possible to discuss with the couple, how to reactivate the partnership sexuality they both long for.

Case Report 13 (Continued)

Often, the syndyastic focus can be limited to few sessions whenever the involvement of the partner is possible and the couple is ready for a change in their relationship. This can be achieved by helping the couple to realize that:

- It is possible to talk about a sexual problem,
- Their difficulties are in good hands and that there is no need to be ashamed of anything,
- The new information might help to readjust their view on the world of sexuality,
- They can help themselves by broadening their sexual behaviour repertoire, attaining new alternatives for themselves to fulfil their (mutual) needs for closeness, caring and acceptance,
- By this fulfilment, no matter how difficult the barriers or restrictions might be, self-confidence arises, and
- Coping strategies are now available for cases of possible adverse reactions from the partner, e.g. after surgical interventions with physical impairments like in the case of implementing a stoma or an artificial bladder.

Concluding Couple Session During the couple session it became obvious that the patient's sexual difficulties were experienced quite differently by his wife. Misunderstandings were cleared impressively. In fact, the wife described how she had always thought, throughout the whole marriage, that she could never satisfy him sexually, because she knew about his frequent masturbation practice; he, on the other hand, had always assumed that she took him for an insufficient lover because of his premature climaxes. She used this opportunity to explain, how important for her non-genital practice as part of sexuality was. This again, was quite relieving for him, because he, too, loved to just lie close to her and to "feel her closeness". So, both declared that they had been taking wrong attitudes of the partner for granted and that improved sexual communication is to be acquired by mutual syndyastic fulfilment. They resolved for the future to talk about their sexual wishes, to create opportunities of enjoying these and to do this quite pragmatically, e.g. if they felt like it, to make use of a morning erection.

A further session after 3 months showed that these resolutions were kept. Both appeared quite changed, fresh and alive as a couple. They had revived their mutual sexuality and were very relaxed about enjoying their intimate contact. They had had sexual intercourse several times, in which no erectile disorder had arisen and the man did not experience his early orgasm as premature at all, even though he did not have the feeling of being able to control the arousal progression. Most important was: He was now completely sure that his wife did not mind this. She, herself, was extremely happy about the expansion of the non-coital sex (i.e. changed view on significance of sexual arousal and desire). This way, both experienced appreciation and acceptance in physical closeness, i.e. fulfilment of fundamental needs, and had, thus, found access for themselves to the syndyastic dimension of sexuality.

Shortly after this session the wife wrote a grateful letter to the therapist, expressing her happiness about the revived marital sexuality ("It's a great feeling, to be man and woman again") and she also expressed her surprise about the fact that "a third party could play such an important role in partnership togetherness".

Conclusions This case report shows clearly that the worrying erectile disorder of the man was only to be understood and successfully treatable under the aspect of a biopsychosocial viewpoint on sexuality as well as under consideration of the attachment aspect of sexual disorders which means the syndyastic dimension of sexuality. In this case there was no need for any deep understanding of the life history and the sexual experiences, but most of all awareness to what was troubling both partners and to pick up their need for physical communication—extra-genital and genital. Only by involving the partner, this neediness became evident and the syndyastic fulfilment was made attainable for both.

It must be said, however, that this case was dealing with an ideal course of sexological counselling with a syndyastic focus—in everyday practice this not always proceeds so smoothly. Often, for example, the involvement of the partner is not a simple matter. And even if the partner does come along, the conversation with the couple might find one or both of the couple unable to cope with the idea of the "reorganisation" of the sexual relationship, especially when different inhibiting factors exist at the same time, e.g. an erectile disorder due to a radical prostatectomy and impairment of physical mobility with pain in certain positions. But also in such cases it should always be attempted to improve the requirements for the fulfilment of psychosocial needs in both partners by applying the syndyastic focus. Very often, talks about male myths and anxiety caused by a bad conscience (masturbation is sometimes seen as betrayal of the partner, sometimes even as immoral) are just as helpful as a survey concerning wishes of closeness and how to make them happen.

During sexological counselling, there are often a great number of influencing factors on the biological, psychosocial and sexual level, which are all important to take note of, but on the other hand must not concentrate the attention of the therapist in such a way as to neglect the syndyastic focus. Such factors are:

- Possible effects of a primary disease (e.g. hypertonia, condition after heart attack) and connected anxieties.
- Possible effects of medication (e.g. beta receptor antagonists, often suspected of causing disorders of sexual function and this is often given as an explanation by patients.
- Physical changes due to ageing.
- Change of social status (e.g. retirement).
- Dynamics of sexual myths ("a man has to be ready at all times").
- Wrong ideas about the needs and expectations of the (female) partner combined with feelings of guilt, not to be able to live up to them.
- Similar wrong ideas in the (female) partner, also combined with feelings of guilt and insufficiency (not to be good enough as a woman, etc.).

- Lacking opportunities of mutual correction concerning misjudgements due to communication barriers.
- Chronification with increasing psychological stress and development of self-reinforcement mechanisms such as failure anxieties and performance pressure—these could lead to maintaining the symptoms.

6.2.3 Sexuality and Partnership in the Elderly

Particularly in older age with its various burdens, general changes and losses, not least the imminence of life's end, signals of love and caring, esteem, concern, closeness and security—also in the non-verbal language of sexuality—are more than ever vital and directly responsible for feelings of self-respect and self-esteem, attitude to meaning of life and happiness. Accordingly, the grounds for relationships in older men and women are such as the desire of not wanting to be alone, living love and companionship, caring and being cared for, with or without sexuality, living apart or together, having a long-term partnership or marriage, or affairs with different partners—all kinds of relationship modes are possible and practiced in reality (Zank 1999). Limitations are set, most of all, by the unequal ratio of women to men. Biopsychosocially based sexual medicine wants to feature the salutogenic potential of a communicative sexuality and to keep it available for a lifetime, making it necessary to also work on questions concerning sexuality during older age.

This is even more important, seeing that the subject of sexual life in the elderly undergoes stronger taboos than the demographic development and sexological facts might imply: People do not only grow older, but they are fit and healthy far longer, keeping their sexual interests and fantasies awake (but old prejudices and educational encumbrances may also remain active). Sexual functions generally age slower than other physical functions.

Basically it can be said that there is no such thing as old-age sexuality. Every individual remains a sexual being and grows old with his or her lifelong mode of sexuality, regardless of his or her sexual orientation: A person who has been living a fulfilled sexual life will want to keep it that way, for others, age could be a welcome excuse to put an end to this chapter in life as soon as possible.

Wherever possible and desired, sexual activity (within a partnership and/or autoerotic) remains a part of life into old age (empirically, at any age, coitus and masturbation are more frequent in men). There are, however, "normal" age-related changes as well as effects in the case of co-morbidity: In men, sexual reaction usually gradually becomes slower and weaker.

The amount of seminal fluid and the intensity of sexual feeling decreases. Erections may be less strong and not as long lasting, the nightly and morning spontaneous erections may decrease, refractory time may be prolonged. This would make stronger and more direct stimulation necessary. Despite the gradual hormonal conversion (in contrast to women), sexual functions in men are more inclined to disturbances than in the aging women and their self-confidence is (too) closely linked to their "potency".

In both genders, sexual activity has a positive influence on the functions: "Use it or lose it" was a key phrase by Masters and Johnson regarding sexuality in older age.

Women experience a drastic hormonal conversion during their menopause and the end of fertility with consequences on body image (relocation of fat distribution) and questioning their self-esteem (still attractive and loved?). It may come to problems such as decrease of vaginal elasticity (perhaps irritable bladder and correlated problems during coitus), atrophy of the vaginal tissue, lack of lubrication fluid, less orgastic contractions as well as changes in skin and general sensitivity in the breast and an altogether slowing down of sexual reaction, making a longer duration of coitus necessary. Such changes may result in hypoactive sexual desire disorders, disorders of sexual arousal, dyspareunia and disorders of sexual orgasm. Desire, arousal and orgastic capability are influenced more by psychosocial partnership factors than by hormonal conditions. At the same time, disorders may take place in the older person of the partnership, so that sexual activity in the couple is reduced. In any case, talks with both partners and within the couple or, in the case of a single person, with this individual, to avoid misinterpretations of situations are extremely important (women tend to "blame" themselves, men believe not to be a good lover without full erectile function, both retreat from the partner(ship)).

As yet, much too little attention is given to this indication for sexological counselling (and optional medicational, apparative or surgical support) here in order to maintain life quality, if the border between help and forced helpfulness is not overstepped. This kind of counselling would also be effective for relatives and nursing home personnel in order to promote a greater understanding of sexuality, particularly in the elderly.

In institutions, it is generally necessary to support development of more structures in the sense of architectural improvements, house rules, daily routine schedules, protection of privacy, etc. allowing for more intimacy in "senior residences".

Reaching a certain age does, however, also offer new chances for an active sexual life, e.g. larger amount of freedom in life organization and a greater amount of intimacy through long years of closeness, more spontaneity due to lack of contraception or fear of pregnancy, longer coitus duration before orgasm, vitalization of the cardiovascular system, activation of the "syndyastic system" (hormone/neurotransmitter release), prevention of atrophic processes, strengthening of the immune system, general biosocial harmonization and "well-being" as a lifestyle reality.

Case Report 14
A Brief Sexological Counselling with a Couple Aged 70 and 72
A vital, fit-looking couple with silver hair visits the urological out-patient department in order to have the vacuum pump explained to them. The man speaks about the loss of his potency (meaning, in fact, erection capability) 2 years before, probably in connection with his heart disease. According to the surgeon, the corporacavernosa of the penis "were damaged".

Some months later, he has heart transplantation surgery and is released to go home 4 weeks later. Erection capability does not return within the following 2 years, he does, however, now and again perceive slight erections during the night time and in the mornings. Sometimes, with manual help by his wife, these would enable coitus lying on the side. Implantation of a penis prosthesis does not come into consideration due to the ongoing immune suppressive therapy.

The couple has a very positive attitude towards sexuality, is keen on a mutual sexual life, the wife as much as the husband, and both claim not to have any other problems within the partnership. They consider sexuality as a passionate form of communication, both radiating optimism and happiness. Issues concerning sexuality after heart transplantation surgery are discussed, the significance of sexual communication emphasized and on this basis the vacuum pump and its working mechanisms and capabilities are explained and demonstrated.

It is known from literature that long-term use of the device (in approximately 25 %) may have positive effects on returning erection capability and actually, a certain training effect could take place. Both partners can come to terms with the idea of utilizing the device, the wife would help "hands on"; they would purchase it and report their experience by telephone.

After 8 weeks, the husband calls to say that he has been using the device for 5 weeks, 15–20 minutes daily for training purposes and that he is quite satisfied with it. He wants to "train my penis" without involving the penis ring and explains cheerfully that the nightly and morning erections are completely restored to their previous state. During spontaneous sexuality they find the device interfering, so his wife stimulates him manually and intercourse takes place in the described manner (lying on the side) and he already has a feeling of steady improvement. His report sounds very enthusiastic and motivated—the couple is satisfied with this solution.

It is more of academic interest, whether or not these statements can be objectified. According to the Masters and Johnson sentence "use it or lose it" there is some credibility in that and the psychosocial effect of daily "penile training sessions" in favour of the own as well as the mutual sexuality is definitely not to be underestimated.

6.3   Syndyastic Sexual Therapy

6.3.1   Goals of Sexual Therapy

As mentioned previously, the general aim of sexual therapy is to enable both partners to satisfy each other's fundamental needs—based on full acceptance—through their sexual behaviour, i.e. their positive sexual communication in partnership. Negative sexual experiences create and sustain sexual disorders which are bound to put strain on a partnership. Here, within the setting of sexological treatment, an understanding of the three dimensions of sexuality and their significance can be combined with well-directed evaluation and open talks about new physical experiences. In this way, partnership intimacy may be revived as a result of newly shared sexual experiences by which intimacy previously experienced might change considerably.

The priority is not to restore sexual function in the first place, the therapeutic aim is to broaden the understanding of sexuality (particularly to appreciate the dimension of attachment), thereby gathering new experiences of (sexual) body communication and improving (sexual) partnership satisfaction on the whole. The option of effective medication or other aids is no contradiction and can be a helpful supplement at times (see Chap. 6.4).

Thus, within the course of therapy, new, mutually agreed upon, intimate experiences for the couple emerge, allocating a new significance of sexuality in a much broader sense. These are no "prescriptions", because it is not possible to "prescribe" anything in a relationship; they are genuine, holistic and consciously lived partnership experiences.

It is quite obvious that, in an existing partnership, the syndyastic focus is most effectively utilized by genuine partner involvement, placing the partnership itself, i.e. the couple, into the centre of attention. Particularly by sexually lustful physical acceptance and intimate closeness elementary needs are likely to be most intensively fulfilled. It is, however, to be noted, that this involves activation of a basically already-existing potential. Something is retrieved and nothing is "added", which also discloses the limits of this treatment method.

Finally, it must be stressed that the syndyastic sexual therapy method is not restricted to certain specialized fields or schools. It merely relies on a basic psychosomatic understanding and the willingness not to project oneself into the role of the objective expert, but to actually concentrate on the syndyastic focus—trusting in the knowledge that improvement of the fulfilment of psychosocial fundamental needs can lastingly affect all other areas of life, health and well-being. As mentioned before, the true motive is clear from the beginning, when a patient or a couple directly consults a sexological therapist. This is by no means the case when, on consulting a specialist or a general practitioner, a causal connection with sexual and/or partnership-related problems is revealed and then understanding of this has to be initiated.

6.3.2 Initial Phase: Motivation for Therapy

In the (quite common) case of a patient/couple being fixated on purely somatic causes it will be crucial not to fall into the *organic or psychological trap*. It would be best to flatly avoid using the often negatively understood term "psychological" causes altogether, e.g.: *You are here as a whole person with a body, a mind and feelings, living human relationships. All these things exist simultaneously and influence each other. Perhaps you are not used to doctors taking all these aspects into account instead of concentrating on the body alone.*

This course will be kept up by asking about "partnerships" instead of only asking about sexuality, usually (mis)understood as genital sexuality—e.g.: ... *everyone needs a place to feel accepted, where somebody cares for you, where you can speak openly, be yourself and feel safe etc.—where is such a place in your life? What is your partnership like? What part does sexuality play within this relationship?*

So, if during a one-to-one conversation the impression is that relationship, partnership and/or sexuality plays a significant part in genesis and continuation of a particular disorder, it will be necessary to motivate the patient to involve the partner and to accept the offer of couple counselling. For example: ... *whatever happens within a partnership concerns both partners and only both together can work on a solution. Both are suffering from this problem and most probably both could use some help. Without your partner it would be like doing things half right from the beginning. What do you think and do you think your partner would agree to come?* If the answer is: *I'm not quite sure* or *my husband/my wife/my friend will definitely not come* it will be necessary to go into the anxiety behind this and also to react to the "invitation", such as: *That would really surprise me. In my experience it is extremely seldom that a partner would refuse this offer—and this in itself would be significant—but how would you put the matter to him/her?* Under some circumstances a dialog involving role play might be encouraging and lead to an acceptable manner of announcement, not allowing for misunderstandings such as sounding like *a legal summons to a trial.* In any case, success very much depends on the convincing manner and resoluteness of the therapist. It could be that unconsciously the patient and the therapist do not want a "third party" to join their relationship; in that case he/she would most likely refuse participation. At this stage of discussion the question could arise, whether an upcoming therapy should be carried out personally or if the case should (or needs to) be passed on to a specialist? Very often, this question remains academic, because the patient/the couple have already inspired confidence: *If we/I do decide to do it, then only with you.*

No matter whether in individual sessions or sessions together with the couple, from the beginning the conversation should be run like the most natural thing in the world. If things such as inhibitions or shame, uncertainty, feelings of guilt or embarrassment are in the air, this should directly be addressed, e.g.: *From my experience I know quite well, that it can be a huge effort to talk to a third party about personal and intimate issues. Many people believe that only they themselves have such problems, in reality, these are quite common, but not many try to solve them professionally. Therefore, making the effort of asking for help is a sign of caring and looking out for a continuation of the partnership.*

If it is a "couple session" from the start, it begins before the first words are spoken with the perception of the partners' interaction, their performance, e.g. *How do both enter the room (overall impression, body language, facial expression, etc). Who leads the way, opens the door, assists at taking off the coat, looks for a seat, is seated first? What is the sitting position like: next to one another, opposite each other or across the corner?* A reply to the question, *Where should we be seated?* could be like *wherever you like,* noting that the therapist takes his seat after the couple. A table with four chairs or several freely placed chairs are more appropriate than a small sofa, on which the couple would be forced to sit next to each other. (No need to say that the therapist should not hide behind his desk.) Which one of them begins the conversation, do the individuals look at each other or do both just look at the therapist, do they interrupt each other's speech?, etc.

If a patient has been able to motivate his/her partner to take part in a session, quite a lot of movement has come into the partnership, even if it might seem as if someone "uninvolved" has just come along to support his/her partner. Generally, men are more inhibited when it comes to discussing relationship issues, therefore the positive decision to come along deserves recognition such as: *good of you to come—I expect it wasn't so easy?*

After an open invitation to the couple to start with whatever seems to them to be most important, the therapist should chose the right moment to define his own role, e.g.:

Maybe I should say something about my role in our talks, so that from the beginning you do not misinterpret it or get the wrong idea. I am neither judge nor referee, who makes decisions about which one of you is in the right. This is not about judgments or guilt, it is about causes and the understanding of how things are connected. It is also not my job to solve your problems, you need to do that yourselves and I can try to help you do so. I am not the expert on your relationship, so you won't be getting any advice from me, only suggestions/ideas. It will be crucial to put the ideas we develop here and whatever you "prescribe" to yourself to work in the outside world. I will not take sides with either one of you, but will step in for both of you and your partnership, as long as it is in your intention. Should one of you still have a feeling of partiality on my part or coalition being built up, please don't hesitate to refer to it.

The setting favoured by Masters and Johnson (1966) in which clients, as a couple, sit opposite a therapist-couple avoids the last-mentioned problems, but is very seldomly conducted. Usually—depending on the gender of the therapist—one male and two females or one female and two males will sit opposite one another and—again—it is important to ask, if there is any suspicion of coalitions or worries of any kind.

On the other hand, usurpation efforts on the part of the patient/couple have to be immediately opposed. Statements like: *Doctor, see for yourself. ..., what do you say to that?, you have to confess, I'm right... tell my partner, he doesn't believe me...,* etc. could be retorted by saying: *Are you looking for an ally?* Or: *You want to make me a referee, which I am not!* Or: *What would it mean to you if I were to say you were right, or you were wrong?* Or: *I can't take that off your shoulders, but this would be a great opportunity to tell your partner personally what is really bothering you. Do try to make him/her understand and perhaps we can find out, what it is all about.*

In such situations it is important not to directly answer the questions reflex-like with regard to content, similar to one would in organic medicine, but to keep out of the content level and to stay on the meta or interpretation level, in order to be able to continue work with both parties.

Often, right at the beginning there is the situation of having to directly refer to anxieties and to disperse these, for instance the fear of being given the death sentence for the relationship or the inevitability of a separation. The anxious question: *According to your experience, do we still have a chance?* is often put forward already in the first session. It has to be taken up on, but must not be dealt with in a direct way, for example: *You're asking me?—You know yourself and your relationship much better than I know you, how much chance do you yourself think you have?* Or: *Whether or not you do have a chance depends on, whether or not you give yourself one and you would probably not be here if you didn't, right?* Or, for example in particular function disorders: *I can generally say, that in the case of these disorders there are statistically very good chances of success, but statistics say nothing about an individual case. So I can't say whether you belong to the 80 % success rate or to the other 20 %—this you decide yourself.*

Before therapy begins, however, it is inevitable to negotiate the practical procedure in detail and to clarify the essential parameters, because it is crucial for success of therapy to comply with these. In accordance, for the whole duration of therapy, both partners need to be able to concentrate on each other and the new common experiences. Therefore, external sexual relationships are incompatible with these requirements and any desire for having children should not be a key issue.

Generally, this is easily conveyed, because the time period of a therapy is seldom more than 3–6 months. Furthermore, there would be no point in beginning with a syndyastic sexual therapy, if the couple has not enough opportunity to gather intimate experiences with one another. This needs to be seen as a specific obligation prior to therapy by both partners.

In same-gender partnerships there are insofar modifications to consider, as the typical gender differences of sexual behaviour (see Beier et al. 2005) in the partners very probably do not occur complementarily. Therefore, it could, perhaps, be expected in a male couple that both partners show a higher willingness for occasional sexual contacts and for them the general significance of infidelity may allow for a relaxed reaction, thus not questioning the syndyastic fulfilment within the partnership. But exactly this is the determining point: The partnership is in danger, only if the biopsychosocial elementary needs—existent in both genders, independent of their sexual orientation—are frustrated. The syndyastic dimension of partnership can, however, be strengthened in many ways, namely always by giving the partner the feeling that he/she is appreciated, taken seriously and accepted and when they feel mutually secure in each other's company. If an external sexual contact does authentically not mean destabilization (which is practically never the case in two-gendered couples), then the syndyastic experience is not threatened.

Nevertheless, sexual communication is a particularly intensive opportunity of finding syndyastic fulfilment and this also applies to one-gendered couples, in which trust in mutual intimacy usually reaches a deeper experience level than one found in occasional external sexual contacts.

6.3.3 New Experiences with Intimacy: The Practical Approach

The central goals of the *syndyastic sexual therapy* are: internalizing the syndyastic dimension of sexuality and the new view on meaning of sexual arousal and desire. This can only be achieved through plausible self-evident experiences by the patient(s)/the couple, enabling them to experience their intimacy as an effective opportunity of fulfilling their fundamental needs for closeness, appreciation and acceptance. That is the only way to change their former "view on the world of sexuality". It is inevitable that the couple needs to "organize" these new experiences—to "make them happen". It is all about practicing improved physical communication (body language) at certain previously appointed times, which will lead to a new experience. This obviously implies that communication on the partnership level itself has to be improved. This means, the first experiences will often touch on the partnership communication as such. This automatically points out the significance of the time between the therapy sessions in which the patient(s)/couples themselves do the main work concerning the intended change of their situation. They put into effect their own previously made resolutions for meaningful new experiences from one session to the next.

In this respect it can be called a "self-prescribed experience" or a mutually conceived resolution. Here the difference to previous well-known popular terminology becomes obvious—no more "home work", "exercises", "sensuality training" or "prescribed experiences". During the *syndyastic focus* it is exactly *not the therapist* who organizes the experiences for the couple and virtually imposes these upon them, rather, the couple finds an own way of creating opportunities for the fulfilment of fundamental needs and finally their connection to sexual arousal and pleasure. The therapist accompanies the couple along this path. Consequently, a further significant difference to classic sexual therapy emerges as it provides for achieving a final goal (namely the restoration of sexual function(s)) in stages. Those various "preliminary steps" are only "a means to an end", while, according to the syndyastic therapy concept the therapy goals are to be fully reached at any stage: with each new experience, the couple may reach the therapy goal completely—it is the task and the responsibility of the therapist, to convey this adequately.

The process of the following experience steps towards improvement of sexual communication is orientated on the so-called "sensate-focus-practice" (sensuality training according to Masters and Johnson), but receives a new allocation of significance. First, the steps need to be understood and internalized as body language communication, so that from the beginning they are more than a training programme for all sensory functions, they are, as a matter of fact, personal body language communication and encounter. Before this is not fully understood, these experience steps should not be started with.

First Step: Mutual Body Discovery, Omitting Breast and Genitals The agreement, to omit the erogenous zones of breast and genitals from the body language communication as well as to abstain from the (often problematic) intercourse (the so-called ban on intercourse by Masters and Johnson) usually arises and makes sense during the discussion of the concrete situation and is often suggested by the couple themselves. For instance, it gives a woman suffering from hypoactive desire disorder or sexual aversion the necessary security that out of a tender display of affection "nothing more" will arise, but the fulfilment of fundamental needs and that it will not "end in sex". A man with problems of erection or orgasm obtains the security that "he can't go wrong" and doesn't have to worry that again "it won't work". As a rule—as always, there are rare exceptions—the strict abstaining from sexual intercourse is the precondition to make really new experiences on the communicative level which have their value in their own right and should not be degraded to "a step on the ladder up to the real thing".

Second Step: Involvement of the Female Breast Again, in a pleasurable tentative way not aimed at sexual arousal, in the next move the female breast can become involved in the exploring and caressing. In communicative meaning, the attention to this particular zone of femininity can express, e.g. appreciation, attractivity, invitation and the pleasure, being welcome—once again mutual acceptance, not reduced to sex appeal.

Third Step: Involvement of the Genitals In this step, too, the coitus still remains banned, but now the genitals can be included into the playful caressing. By now, for the couple, there should be an understood difference between "purposeful" sexual arousal (with one thing in mind) and "random playfulness" on the level of body language communication, so that exhilarating experiences can be made without erection and/or orgasm. It is extremely important that both partners take joint responsibility for mutually satisfying intimacy (and therefore, e.g. direct the partner's hand to the place they like to be caressed.) This promotes the most important goal of the therapy: internalization of the syndyastic dimension of sexuality.

Interventions to reach the goal of the therapy: internalization of the syndyastic dimension of sexuality:

1. Detailed evaluation of the agreed upon experiences ("exercises") concerning concrete behaviour (what has been done?) and the experience of it (how was it perceived?).
2. Translation of the experiences as an expression of fulfilled fundamental needs. For example: One of the partners felt very "close" or especially "accepted" by the other while caressing. As it were, "closeness" and "acceptance" had specifically been felt, had happened, made happen by behaviour. The most important thing is to make this obvious for the couple.
3. Principally, this can be enacted on all experience levels, as well as sexual behaviour in a narrower sense (e.g. genital acceptance, being close, being open) so that the reaching of this goal of therapy can (and should) be pointed out from the start.

Fourth Step: Teasing and Arousal If the couple focuses on the topic of desire (which may be present from the beginning) lust is also connected to the dimension of attachment, because it arises on the basis of mutual acceptance. This way it is easy to explain to the patients that they can experience a syndyastic enhancement of their passion respectively a sensual–orgastic enhancement of their partnership. From a therapeutic point of view it is all about connecting the dimension of desire with the syndyastic dimension, meaning a changed view on and significance of sexual arousal and desire.

Interventions to reach the goal of therapy: "New meanings for sexual arousal and desire":

1. Dealing with sexual arousal and desire will (deliberately) become an issue in the further course of the "exercises".
2. But this now happens on the basis of the internalized attachment-oriented dimension of sexuality: Both partners are aware of the fact that they are mutually fulfilling their need for acceptance, closeness, etc. through intimacy.
3. Passionate desire, therefore, is intertwined with the dimension of attachment, because it has arisen on the basis of mutual acceptance. A practical example: The husband reports about his enthusiasm concerning his sexual arousal. When questioned about the significance of his wife in this context ("Which role did your wife actually play?" or: "Could it have been any other woman?) makes her specific role obvious.
4. By asking questions such as "What does that mean concerning the experience of desire?" and "What does it mean in terms of partnership experience?" the quality of partnership and desire can be appreciated as two mutually strengthening aspects. The man with his desire is accepted by the woman; he can have the feeling of being accepted in his sexual identity as a male and vice versa, i.e. the woman will be enhanced in her sexual identity as a female by his desire for her alone.

Fifth Step: Non-Demanding Coitus The next step could add sexual intercourse, but still with the intention of getting to know one's own reaction better and to make new experiences with the partner, in order to, for instance consciously experience the body language messages during the intercourse like in "slow motion", stripping off anxieties, gaining security, etc. They have mutually agreed to relax after penetration. So, this non-demanding intromission (sometimes termed "quiet vagina") is not about spontaneous complete coitus. This step can also be applied in the treatment of orgasm praecox (see Chap. 4.1, 4.3).

Sixth Step: Spontaneous, Whole Coitus. Here, the connection between the syndyastic system and the system of desire should be so stable that it remains internalized, even when not thinking about it all the time. Sexual desire should now be consciously experienced in the context of fulfilled fundamental needs and be therefore more intensive and more intimate as a whole. Sex and love should no longer be in any way separated in the partner, but be moulded into one. Only in this entity, desire can really develop freely, as long as the communication is experienced as authentic.

As in classical sexual therapy, special techniques such as "stop-start" or "squeeze" can be integrated into syndyastic sexual therapy, but need to be understood and utilized on the basis of the treatment's focal point, the attachment dimension of sexuality. The woman might stimulate the penis to near climax but would need the response from the partner, in order to interrupt at the right moment; this only works, if, on the basis of their relationship understanding, she really feels involved and not just as being used similar to a random physiotherapist.

It needs to be emphasized that this programme must never be prescribed in the way of "cooking recipes", but can ever individually and by involving the couple be generously varied (see detailed case reports in Chap. 6.5).

The conclusive summary (see box) once again shows the different steps of the *syndyastic sexual therapy*, which must not lead to the wrong conclusion, that the therapy goal is only reached at the final step, because every step bears the (potential of) therapeutic goals already in itself and is able to express an improved sexual and partnership contentedness. Putting it another way: the first three steps preferably deal with the syndyastic level of sexuality and mutual partnership interaction, while steps four to six give an opportunity of experiencing the syndyastic enhancement of desire as well as specifically experiencing the passionate-orgasic enhancement of the partnership itself.

Syndyastic sexual therapy: possible steps for improvement of body language communication:

1. Involvement of the whole body (from head to toe), but not the genital region and the female breast (agreed upon abstaining from intercourse).
2. Involvement of the female breast in the exploring and caressing, but again in a pleasurable discovering way and not aimed at sexual arousal.
3. Involvement of the genital region (the coitus ban is still valid) in playful caressing.
4. Playful handling of arousal and checking out the own curve of arousal, where it still should not come to orgasm (pleasurable experiences can be made without erection and/or orgasm).
5. Non-demanding coitus.
6. Sexual intercourse.

Note Every one of these possibilities to gain "new experiences" already bears the (potential of) treatment goals in itself, because an improved sexual and partnership contentedness can be expressed and reached at any step. At no stage must the couple have the impression that the real goal can only be reached at steps 5 or 6.

Conducting syndyastic sexual therapy in an elderly couple works just as well as in a younger one (see the following case report).

Case Report 15 Twenty-years-old C.O. is of Turkish descent, since the age of 5 grown up in Berlin, where he graduated from high school and is now studying at the university. He reports having orgasm praecox, prevalent since the beginning of having socio-sexual relationships (i.e. lifelong type), while during masturbation being "quite well" able to control arrival of sexual climax (i.e. situational type). With his 1 year younger German girlfriend, just graduating from school, he ejaculates at the very moment of trying to enter her vagina. Their way of coping is to wait until he is "ready for a second try", then he would not reach climax so soon and his girlfriend would sometimes have time to build up arousal herself or (rarely) be able to reach climax, as well.

He is very much in love with his girlfriend, although she, as a German, is not allowed to go to his home—his family is very traditional and would only accept his future wife as a visitor to their home. He is just as frustrated as his girlfriend, sees himself as "unmanly" ("a loser") and has bought "lots of literature" about masturbatory practice, but this has not helped in intimate situations at all.

In the context of a syndyastic sexual therapy of ten sessions, which the girlfriend was prepared to take part in—considering the perspective of their future relationship—both were quite soon capable of sharing mutual intimate experiences without anxieties. He experienced the fact of not having to concentrate on his penis, or arousal level or any possibly oncoming sexual climax as "extremely relaxing": In the (particularly important) first phase of therapy these issues take a back seat in the context of sensuality training, explicitly to strengthen the awareness for the attachment dimension of sexuality ("syndyastic focus") at this point.

During this process it became obvious that especially the girlfriend profited immensely by this new point of view, while C.O. himself saw "long duration capability" as his goal to success and had more difficulties in coming to terms with a different allocation of meaning. During playful handling of arousal, namely building-up arousal and let it fade away, he did profit greatly and said himself that his "point of view" was now "different", so that in her company he seemed more relaxed which was rated as success. At the end of the therapy, vaginal sexual intercourse was no problem and the time span from penetration to climax was described as adequate by both of them.

6.3.4 Detailed Exploration

During this kind of work with the couple it is important right from the start (as by the way also in the partnership) to pay attention to details and nuances and particularly to the significance it has for each individual of the couple. In addition to the usual (macro) anamnesis, there has to be the micro anamnesis, the inquiring into and asking for elaboration of the slightest details: *What exactly was that like? How did you experience it? What exactly was normal about it, good or dreadful? What did it mean to you in that situation at that time?* Doing this, it is not primarily about working through "psychotherapeutic pathways", it is about the "syndyastic focus" on the violated (or fulfilled) elementary needs of being acknowledged, desired and respected, feeling accepted, trusting, experiencing closeness and being sheltered, etc. Which of these needs have been frustrated and what kind of significance have they obtained during the biography of this person? At the same time, the partner will be asked questions such as: *Is that the way you saw it too? Are you agreeing cognitively or emphatically? Were you aware of the significance for your partner?* Often, one partner (normally the man) uses facts for argument, the other partner is on a level of feelings and meanings, which results in them not really talking to each other and the whole argument escalates.

Being uncertain of what action to take in case of uncontrollable disputes is what keeps many doctors from doing couple sessions. However, it is not at all the therapist's job to settle such arguments, rather to observe and raise questions. For instance: *Do your disputes always go like this? Is this typical of what it's like at home? Was it ever any different and how did you manage that?* Or something like: *How would you feel, if you were spoken to like that? What do you expect to achieve by it? Do you think you will be successful?*

Equally disturbing are long pauses where both are silent. These must be given room and endured for the patient's/couple's contemplation and thought tracking. There is, of course, the possibility of asking about their significance. In this case, own ideas could indicate a diagnostic direction of the patient's/couple's state of mind and could be, reflectively, offered as a question (see box).

Perceiving One's Own Feelings in the Context of the Syndyastic Sexual Therapy

- Consciously reflecting one's own feelings instead of (re)acting in an un-reflected spontaneous way.
- Can these feelings be clearly named, are they understandable or are they contradictory, vague, not concrete?
- In what way are they "my own" feelings connected closely to my own personality/ life history/present situation—and how far are they induced by the patient/the couple and what might this reveal about his/her/their situation?

In certain cases, micro-anamnestic investigation, especially concerning sexual intimacy, might be in need of explanation, for instance: *I do hope you understand that I am not asking out of personal curiosity, but it is most important to really understand the situation in its significance, especially as it can make things a lot clearer for yourself/and your partner.*

In the case of hypoactive sexual desire, for instance appropriate questions might be: *What is it you yourself would enjoy doing?* Or: *What is it exactly, that you don't feel like, what is it you are too tired for? Can you say what's behind it? For you, where does love end and where does sex start? What does love and sex have to do with one another? What are their differences? What is their common ground?*

Here it might be helpful to insist, for instance: *Did I understand you correctly? Are you saying that. ...?* Or: *Couldn't that also be understood differently, such as. ...?* Or: *Am I wrong or do I hear a certain undertone, which might mean that. ...?*, etc.

This gives the therapist a chance to improve the general communication by playing a role model. Often there are positive things to be acknowledged and successes to be emphasized: *You state this incidentally, but you know it is not to be taken for granted..., a great success..., reason to be pleased. ...*

Sometimes only negative things are expressed: *There is no connection between us any more, the relationship is at an end.* This, of course, may be the case and has to be accepted, but not without questioning it: *... and is that the reason for you both being here together? You might have gone straight to a lawyer for a divorce petition?* Or: *For you, the fire has gone out, but do you think there might be some glowing embers under the ashes that might be turned into flame? And if so, how might we go about it?* Of course, it is not for the therapist to decide such questions, nor to mend the relationship or to separate it. That is something only the couple themselves can decide, but the final mature decision should be well founded and close to reality. This goal is not going to be achieved, if opinions of the couple or one of the partners are too easily and not critically agreed to. After all, the consent to doing a session as a couple is in itself a therapy contract, so decision-making should be given thought, discussion and time. In the final session of a successfully experienced couple therapy, the answer to the question "what helped you most" was "the fact that you did not give up on us".

6.3.5   Syndyastic Sexual Therapy with Patients Suffering from Disorders of Sexual Preference

Clinical experience shows that disorders of sexual preference can often lead to disorders of sexual relationship. In the end, it depends on the question of whether or not the partner would be able to accept these and be able to cope, if fantasy contents were made known to him/her—even, if their execution were not intended. Such uncertainties have the power of destabilizing the syndyastic system so severely that relationships are very difficult to enter into or they put existing ones at great risk (see Chap. 4.4). If, however, a partnership does exist and both partners have an authentic interest in a mutual perspective, the *syndyastic sexual therapy* can be effectual in improving partnership contentment. The following four factors are crucial:

1. *The proportion of the paraphilic pattern in relation to the sexual preference structure*

   It makes a big difference, whether the paraphilic experience affects the whole sexual preference structure, or whether there might be other, non-paraphilic parts, which can be acted out with the partner. For example, in the case of an exclusive masochistic inclination, in which a (gynephilically orientated) man, in order to get sexually aroused, exclusively fantasizes scenes in which he is mutilated by his (female) partner, then there is no way for him to build up a comparable sexually arousing situation any other way with his partner. This, again, would very likely lead to disorders of sexual function (see Chap. 4.1) and would burden the partnership severely, if the partner were kept in the dark and she were not able to understand why there were such difficulties in sexual communication.

2. *Sexual function disorders emerging additionally*
   Just as every disorder of sexual function can be a symptom of another disease (e.g. a disorder of orgasm in multiple sclerosis), there is always the possibility that it might be caused by a paraphilia—precisely because the individual involved does not want to further burden the partnership with his paraphilic stimulus, making him insecure in intimate contact because he fears that the emergence of paraphilic fantasy images would keep him away from his partner, while all he wants is to be close. On the other hand, a functional disorder (e.g. an erectile disorder) is a visually obvious symptom for the partner and generally both partners communicate the wish to change this situation, so that here would be a starting point regarding the therapeutic work, keeping in mind that the explanation about the connection with the feelings of paraphilic experience in itself is an important step within the therapy context (see the case report on syndyastic sexual therapy; Chap. 6.3).

3. *The significance of the paraphilic stimulus within self-experience*
   The fact that an attachment to the paraphilic stimulus can exist (as, e.g. in the case of a fetishistic inclination), affecting the syndyastic experience in such a way that in contact with the stimulus, not only sexually arousing but also psycho-emotionally stabilizing feelings (comparable with those in attachment to another person) are experienced, makes a clear statement concerning the limits of thera-peutic intervention. This applies when the attachment to the paraphilic stimulus (e.g. a fetish) has the same or greater significance for the individual as the attach-ment to a real partner. An especially extreme example for this is the so-called "Cannibal from Rothenburg" whose feelings of attachment were constricted in such a way that he could only experience real "love" towards another person, when this other person was inside of him, whereas other forms of sexual fulfilment were not available, at least not in regard to the desired attachment experience. Diagnos-tically this meant a special form of fetishistic orientation (namely towards male flesh; DSM-IV-TR: 30281; ICD 10: 65.0) without any further psychopathological disorders; see Beier (2007, 2009). However, clinical experience has shown that particularly in fetishistic preference patterns (e.g. diaper fetishism) the attach-ment towards the fetish is so strong that a real partner has little chance to reach this level of significance, so that, from the beginning, there certainly are limits concerning couple-centred intervention.

4. *Ability of self-retraction*
   The significance of the paraphilic pattern in self-experience is not the only therapeutically limiting factor (see above), but also—however, in no way coincident—the ability of self-retraction with regard to the partnership is an issue: In the case of an exclusively paraphilic pattern (e.g. sadism with exclusive and not acceptable stimulus-enhancing content, involving injury or mutilation of the partner) it may be of importance for the individual involved, to aim at

improvement of the attachment contentedness, because for him it may be a resource of life quality which he wants to make use of within a functioning partnership. From a clinical point of view it is striking that this criterion is often found in women with an exclusive type of paraphilia (e.g. a sexual masochism), who much more often emphasise the syndyastic function level in comparison to the dimension of desire. Without doubt there are also women with paraphilias, in whom this is not so, but this is more seldom the case than in men. In addition, an important motivational factor in this context—for men as well—is a feeling of responsibility for existing (or planned) mutual children (see Beier 2010).

A detailed case report referring to a successfully conducted syndyastic sexual therapy concerning paraphilic symptoms is described in Chap. 6.5 (see "Case Report E").

6.4   Integration of Somatic Therapy Options

The integration of somatic options within sexual therapy complies with the biopsychosocial character of sexual dysfunctions. It often makes less-invasive somatic interventions necessary, but could shorten the time period of sexual therapy and improve the compliance and the prognosis of all treatment approaches. It is hardly, however, ever conducted in practice. As in all therapy methods, a combined approach can come up with problems as well as chances. Involvement of somatic options may produce the following problems:

- The patient/the couple might mistake the use of a medication as an uncomplicated "rapid repair" method, which would
- Paralyze the self-healing qualities of the couple and could
- Reduce the motivation to tackle personal or partnership problems.

On the positive side, a combined approach:

- Improves effectiveness and prognosis of the treatment in many patients;
- Conveys to the patient that the therapist takes his worries, often fixated on somatic causes, seriously;
- Enables establishment of an initial working bond and
- In the sense of taking the patient seriously meeting him "from where he is standing" and by this means opening up an approach also to the psychosocial side of things.

Particularly in male patients, practical clinical work in sexual medicine often means having to lead the patient—who usually takes it for granted that his problem is related to physical causes—to understand the psychological burden and partnership-relevant angles and to convince him of the biopsychosocial concept of sexuality.

This can only succeed (or succeed much better) if the therapist is well informed about the advantages and disadvantages of pharmaceutical treatment options (which are—in the sense of the method proclaimed here—an acclaimed part of sexual therapy), discusses them with the patient signalizing readiness to try certain methods,

Table 6.1 Medication as a possible option in sexological treatment. (Rösing et al. 2009)

Substance	Application	Mechanism of action	Symptoms which may make further medication necessary
Yohimbine	Oral	Central alpha-2 antagonist, enforces erection benefit	Erection disorder (no effect in ED with somatic correlation)
Sildenafil, vardenafil, tadalafil	Oral	Selective PDE-5-inhibitor, relaxes smooth cavernous muscle tissue by inhibiting the c-GMP-reduction	Erection disorder
	Intracavernous injection therapy (SKAT), transurethral (MUSE)	Prostanoid, leads to relaxation of smooth muscle tissue	Erection disorder
Lidocaine, prilocaine	Local (glans penis)	Locally anesthetizing, diminishes arousal of the penis	Premature orgasm
Fluoxetine, sertraline, paroxetine, dapoxetine	Oral	Serotonine re-uptake inhibitor, stimulation of sexually attenuating central serotonine receptors	Premature orgasm
Testosterone	Oral, transcutane, intramuscular	Central, stimulates the T-synthesis, release and storage of proerectile neurotransmitters (oxytocin, dopamine, NO), testosterone deprivation leads to apoptosis of the smooth cavernous muscle tissue	Substantiated hypogonadism with effects on appetence and erection

SKAT intracavernous injection therapy, *MUSE* medicated urethral system for erection, *NO* nitric oxide, *T* testosterone, *ED* erectile disorder

if the examination findings suggest this and the patient agrees to go along with this approach. If the therapist succeeds in conveying to the patient that it is not about "withholding" certain somatic options such as self-injection or oral medication, but that he is trying to find out their possibilities and their limits, particularly with reference to the couple-relationship. This way an acceptable working bond can be developed, allowing work on the psychological effects as well as the partnership problems (Table 6.1).

6.5   Detailed Case Reports

6.5.1   Case Report A

Disintegrated Dimensions of Desire and Attachment in Both Partners A 40-year-old engineer is referred by his GP to sexological treatment because of "excessive sexual fantasies", which are endangering his working ability. At first he comes by himself and reports of having "24 hours of sexual fantasies a day", which are so burdening that he is not capable of doing proper work, which greatly worries him. He is easily sexually aroused "by everything". Also, for this reason, he is afraid of losing his wife. He has been married for 18 years; two children have come from this marriage, a 16-year-old son and a 12-year-old daughter. From the beginning, their sexual life was not a satisfying one. No paraphilic patterns could be revealed by in-depth exploration.

His wife had always had a rejective and non-enthusiastic attitude towards sexuality because of abuse experience in her youth, "cuddling is enough for her". She was sexually hardly ever active and could only reach orgasm during masturbation. He watched pornographic films with her to animate her, but she rejected that vehemently.

The more he would sexually pressure her, the more she would withdraw and concentrate on the children. Therefore, 7 years into their marriage, he got involved with a 30-year-old single woman and this affair lasted 5–6 years. He was aware of the fact that this woman was having affairs with other men at the same time. She was sexually fine, but was not good at partnership bonding. He had found "his taste for sexuality" with her, but would never have been able to form a partnership with her. For his wife, discovering this affair was a shock and over a long period of time they had only been holding on to their marriage because of the children. For 3 years now, he has definitely not had any more extramarital contacts. He wants to stay with his wife which is the reason for him to seek counselling.

He had met his wife at sports. She had been the illegitimate child of a single mother of 18 years and had never met her biological father. She had been accepted by her stepfather, but had been the Cinderella of the family and, as the eldest, had been burdened with lots of responsibility and had no self-confidence whatsoever. With respect to sexuality she had said to him: "Sexuality destroyed my life, first my stepfather and then your affair". Now, for the first time, he had talked things over with his wife, everything had been said and currently they were having "a great sex life, where I don't miss a thing". He is quite satisfied and now able to work again: "It's good now, but will it stay that way?" He is worried things could change. He reckons "if the sex is good, the partnership is good, too"—but his wife sees things the other way around! It is agreed upon, that he should ask his wife if she would also take part, so that in a few sessions with the couple the current positive situation can be stabilized.

One week later he returns, bringing along his wife, who confirms, that the current partnership situation is satisfactory. She does, however, report that sex never did work well with them, even when they were 23 years old. For years she had had abdominal pain just thinking about sexual intercourse and alone from looking at his penis she was horrified. She herself establishes the connection to her own abuse and reports how her mother told her, at the age of 10, that of now she would have to sleep in the parents' bedroom. Once, her mother caught her father "on top" of her there. For 5 years now she has been trying to talk to her parents about what happened then, but it was not possible. As a reply to her question, why her mother had not helped her, she just said: "I'm not interested in that, it's not my fault". Because she wanted to know more, her family had turned away from her claiming she had destroyed the family. She used to be a light-hearted person but later she had had nightmares and had known that men were bad and that she herself would never want to have an illegitimate child.

For her husband this recount of the story emotionally leads to understanding, in what way his behaviour deeply affected her. Now she hopes to overcome this disappointment. In reply to the question, what actually is the most important thing to her within the relationship, she states: emotional security. But in reply to the question what sexuality has to do with love she says: "I couldn't really say". The fulfilment of fundamental needs with the help of sexual communication takes time to work out. Together with both partners, steps towards "new experiences" were planned, all except intercourse, and they had time for this until the next appointment in 2 weeks.

Two weeks later: The couple had taken time for one another on several occasions and reported: "It is going well". The woman had felt comfortable "he accepts me, the way I am"; it was fun, too, and they had talked a lot. The man sums up: "I think less often about sex, during the daytime not at all; I can go out on the street without seeing every woman as a sex object and I haven't had stomach aches for quite some time, like I used to every day this state has to be kept up". He is worried that his wife might "not like" him and the whole situation "any more"—I don't want it to come to that. Since he had told his former girlfriend that he was doing fine, she had not talked to him again at all. His wife, too, is still insecure and worried: "Will he leave again? Does he like me? I didn't know much about him and focused on caring for the children." The children notice the positive change as well. The woman says that the daughter was actually relieved when she heard about our reason for coming here. She summarizes the most important changes as being: "The barrier in my head is gone—he gives me a feeling of being fond of me and not just wanting sex" and she adds: "I never hated him". He puts forward: "There would be less divorces if people would try as hard, as we do". What remains is the burdening situation with her parents, on that issue there is still a lot to be taken care of. The current state of her relationship is helping her there. Both hope to maintain this state and want to come to an end of the sessions.

Comments This couple was troubled by the huge personal humiliation caused by many years of the husband's infidelity. The breaking down and separation of the two dimensions of sexuality, attachment and desire, as well as the (for her not acceptable) coarse view on sexuality (pornographic films and expressions not quoted in this report) had obviously been tackled and quite "resolved" before the beginning of the sessions. Sexuality was already "working" better than ever before.

However, the decisive breakthrough—also crucial in the prognostic respect—for both partners came through their extended understanding of sexuality, combining both dimensions, desire and attachment. Both partners managed this by consciously experiencing fulfilment of their fundamental needs, in this case the multidimensional experience of desire. Especially the woman was quite capable of clearly expressing the essentials of her relationship to her husband and what had helped her overcome the old traumatization (barrier in her head), validating the accuracy and coherence of the syndyastic approach, substantiating its therapeutic effectiveness and capability of overcoming even grave injuries.

Even if setbacks should occur, the couple can look back on mutual, extremely satisfying experiences, which they might then relate to, if required.

6.5.2 Case Report B

Desire to Have Children in a Couple with Unconsummated Marriage A young married couple visits the GP's outpatient clinic because of their desire to have children and is referred to sexual therapy. They are farmers, married for 3 years, sexual intercourse had never been experienced together. Right at the beginning of their relationship the young woman told her partner that "she has an inner barrier, and force would not do any good". In a women's magazine she read the advice to insert two fingers into her vagina in order to overcome "the barrier". She had done this once with great effort, but after that never again. After an initially harmonious beginning of their relationship, it has turned to frustration: both are disappointed and bitter. He accuses her of lack of enthusiasm and desire, frigidity, rejection, obsessive cleaning and constant nagging; she reproaches him for lack of appreciation, no praise, criticism of the food, not being empathic. When she complains, he shuts himself off, does not listen and "is gone". She had already been to several different female therapists (talks and breathing exercises) without any success and sees her situation as "rather hopeless". Physically there are no pathological findings, in particular no vaginism. Following their own mutual goal in the sense of a self-prescribed "new experience" (aiming at a less-frustrating atmosphere in their partnership) the couple agrees to generally argue less often and praise one another more up to the next session. For 1 week they are successful without quarrels and joint activities, he helps her more—the atmosphere is quite improved.

Now there is room for family assessments, which make things much more transparent: The husband has eight siblings, among them a brother is suffering from muscle dystrophia. The father—a war veteran with an alcohol problem—died early. In this family of farmers there is not much talking, no praise or obvious appreciation of others—"no room for feelings". There was a lot of fighting—so he "shut himself off".

The wife has a 5 years younger brother, having shared the parents' bedroom with him until the age of ten. She cannot remember anything in particular, but when each got their own rooms she was "terribly scared at night that someone would come and do something to her". Sexuality was taboo and devaluated as "nothing special", scared of becoming pregnant ("don't you dare bring a child home") dominated her socio-sexual contact conduct—"pressuring boys had no chance with me". At the age of 15, she touched an erected penis for the first time and was "terribly shocked: what is that?" "The penis is too large, if only it were smaller!" Her emotions, whenever sexuality was concerned: "somebody is telling me, you shouldn't, don't do that!" ("From the bellybutton downward I am dead").

Although there is enough material, even in this very [compressed] excerpt, for a classical psychotherapeutic approach here, syndyastic sexological treatment trusts the healing power of fulfilled fundamental needs within the dimension of attachment (syndyastic focus).

Therefore, "new experiences" on issues of praise, approval, being taken seriously, support ("sometimes I feel like an employee"), attention and affection as well as their body language communication with more or less success are made and talked about.

These talks were very helpful and there were weeks without fighting with more closeness and affection: "So I immediately forgot my anger, I hope he continues being so good to me". In former times, she had been troubled by penis aversion. She might have said in angry disputes: "I'm going to cut your penis off!", now it is: "No, not really—I might still need it" and her husband reacted: "If she doesn't want to cut it off any more, there is nothing for me to worry about, is there?"

But therapies based on theories about castrating women and castration anxieties in men would not be in a position of overcoming these barriers as radical as the direct experience of closeness and warmth (he warms her bed, so it gets "warmer" within their relationship), trust, loyalty and the feeling of security. Neurobiological explanations about the aggression-reducing, harmonizing and attachment-enhancing benefit of oxytocin can compare with the real experience just as little.

During the eighth therapy session the husband happily talked about 3 weeks without quarrels despite straining work and his wife, equally pleased, about an "extremely huge step" for her: without any preparation she was easily able to insert two fingers into her vagina without any pain. "Why did that work so well?" The answer is speculative. Fact is, that her internal barriers, her anger due to violation of fundamental needs in the partnership and the resulting rejection and estrangement from her husband during therapy (8 sessions in 2 5 months) had changed so much for the better, that a physical expression of internal barriers became obsolete. At the same time, step by step the negatively burdened sexuality and sexual passion gained a new meaning as an especially intensive expression of the newly experienced closeness and togetherness. At this point (after having talked about anxieties concerning pregnancy and birth as well as options of contraception) the couple wanted to finish the therapy and to do further steps on their own, what had to be respected as being an authentic wish of the couple.

Follow-up assessment after 16 years: The wife, after questioning, reported that everything had developed well, normal sexual experiences were natural and they had had three children in the meantime.

6.5.3 Case Report C

Hypoactive Sexual Desire Disorder and Dyspareunia A 32-year-old woman from a small town in a rural area is advised by her GP, who is treating her for pressure pain above the heart and complaints concerning spinal pains, to make an appointment. It concerns her unsatisfying sexual life, she has no feelings of desire and experiences pain during sexual intercourse. The gynecologist results are normal. It is agreed upon that she and her husband will come after completion of her physiotherapy (time problem) for an initial session.

First Session This couple in their thirties make a good impression, looking well and attentive, mutually respectful in their conduct. They have been married for 9 years with three children, the youngest just being one year old.

The woman is the first child of a large family, her father a person of authority: "Whenever he said anything, that was enough". She describes herself as having been brought up "strictly Roman Catholic", the family lived in their religious faith, sexuality was rarely an issue, but it was clear that pre-marital intercourse is forbidden and that reproduction was the reason for sexuality. Nevertheless, two of her sisters were already pregnant at the time of their wedding, which was held against the family by the relatives. She describes her childhood as quite normal, no hints of any sexual traumatization. For herself, religion is a huge and important issue. She had taken on lots of tasks: Alongside her own family she was taking care of her mother-in-law, who was living in the same house, sustained her more than 80-year-old parents and additionally worked in the office of the parish. Her husband is her "first man" and "otherwise" they got along quite well.

The husband has a technical vocation, makes a very solid impression, but at home feels to be between two women and suffers a great deal from the unsatisfying sexual situation. His religious beliefs are not so strict and he says his wife, whom he otherwise cherishes, is "quite extreme" in this matter. The wife complains that generally there is not enough talking going on, particularly "it is not possible to talk about religion—that is a great deficit". Also, her husband is not affectionate enough, only for sexual intercourse there is some "targeted tenderness". She had had great expectations regarding her wedding night and was extremely disappointed: It was supposed to "be easy and good", instead of that it had unexpectedly hurt and turned out to be quite difficult. In the 9 years since then, "it had only felt good a few times". Subtle aggression is palpable.

This couple is worked through the significance of basic human needs, the importance of communication and introduced to a new angle on sexuality (general principles of the syndyastic focus). Both are keen on improving verbal and non-verbal communication, i.e. more talks and visible affection and are seriously set on trying this up to the next session. The couple's behaviour is balanced and authentically interested in one another as well as in the relationship, which makes a positive prognosis likely.

Second Session (2 Weeks Later) It did not go well. Showing affection and being together were fine, "but does it always have to end with that?" The wife reports of having a bad conscience, as soon as she notices an erection in her husband—but when it comes to intercourse "there is nothing pleasant for myself in that, only that he is happy. Penetration hurts". The therapist's question whether the fact also hurts, that it is only a physical but not completely emotional act is immediately answered in the affirmative. The woman feels spiritually separated from her husband, because she cannot talk to him about religion. On the other hand, she has come to realize that she can only be tender towards him when he is ill, more or less a feeling of pity. These experiences help to deepen the conviction of how important it is to feel acceptance as a whole person and how disturbing it can be to be ignored or left out of certain fields, which are of importance for the partner. In those cases, sexuality can only partly fulfil its syndyastic function. Therefore, the couple wants to try not to exclude any issue at all during their conversations. At the same time, their "togetherness" is to be quite deliberately aimed at their mutual pleasure, whereby they agree upon excluding intercourse, in order to be able to give undivided attention to body language communication without fear of anxieties.

Third Session (1 Week Later) The husband rated the mutual experiences as very positive, it was fun. His wife, too, had a good time, in the mornings better than in the evenings, because then she felt "safer". "Skin to skin is a lovely feeling" and "best of all was stroking my face". She had never told him, that she had not liked touching his penis. She had had no images of a penis, her husband's was the first she had ever seen—then she suddenly remembers a scene with an exhibitionist in a train. This opened up to a discussion about the new perspective on genitals and sexual intercourse as organs of communication and the physical side of satisfying fundamental needs, owning up that "heart and soul" do agree, but there were still bad feelings about it hurting. She had also been able to speak a little to her husband about religion. She had felt a slight touch of desire herself. "I would so love it to change, but I just cannot believe it, just like that—just by trying?" At the same time, she hesitates: "Would 14 days to the next session be too long?"

The currently made experiences are discussed and it is decided to repeat these and, if they wish, to expand these towards sexual arousal and desire, but always in the light of the new perspective.

After a week, the wife cancels the next session by telephone because she is complaining of nausea and stomach pains (!). She gives a short report that her husband is losing patience, reproaches her and claims to have given up hope—"but for me it's going too fast". Seeing that she is longing for change, she wants to make use of the time.

Fourth Session (1 Week After the Telephonic Conversation) Several times during the past week, the couple has spent time together in the arranged way, but obviously their problem and the pressure of solving it at last has overlayed the originally aimed at—healing—experience. The wife felt no sexual desire (which was not the issue after all!): "I don't miss anything—I only have a bad conscience because of him." And: "We have not discovered the reason yet". "Even touching the penis is not comfortable, not the slack penis, but the erected penis is frightening, it is so hard and hurts". There is no association to any experiences in the past, but all already-verbalized complaints are repeated and made an issue of once more: The disappointment of the wedding night about the pain and the difficulties. Anxieties, feelings of fear and tenseness are obvious and palpable. "That it was supposed to be fulfilling for myself as well. . . I never thought about it that way." She speaks of cramps during menstruation, of not having taken the pill for religious reasons, how important faith and "purity" was, which she did not want to lose before marriage. The contrast to the new concept becomes obvious. Again she refers to her taciturn father as a person of respect, with whom she was unfortunately not able to speak the way she would have wanted to. For her "being able to talk" is very important.

Her husband listens to her more, "understands" her better and really tries to be acceptingly empathic. She realizes the fact that he is not the "born speaker", which makes her value his efforts. A further session is arranged for 2 weeks later. It is suggested that she experiments with inserting her finger into the vagina, taking notice of her feelings, perhaps pain, in doing that.

Fifth Session For a start, the husband reports alone (because his wife is a little delayed), that he does not understand the whole thing because the initiative of marriage came from her. He, however, is sure to be the right partner for her and blames religion, "you have to be patient". But he admits to having lived sexuality quite apart from tenderness and "intimacy in mutual communication by talking" and has become aware of the fact that he is playing the part of the taciturn father-in-law: What he says, goes, he is the person of respect, but he is unreachable and distant which excludes the fulfilment of fundamental needs such as being accepted, feeling closeness and security and altogether an all-round experience of sexual communication. So, he has been trying to pay more attention to his wife's feelings and showing his own feelings more openly and describes a positive change of climate. His wife (having arrived in the meantime) confirms this: "The whole atmosphere is more pleasant, there is more tenderness and we talk more". She is experiencing more closeness in the partnership and wants to undertake more mutual activities. Inserting several fingers into her vagina caused no problems, no pain. Sexual intercourse had not taken place as yet, but they are both open for a chance of doing so. Past feelings of hopelessness have made room for careful optimism. A further session is arranged for 2 weeks later.

Sixth Session The couple walks in, obviously relaxed and reports of a "surprisingly lovely", fulfilling intercourse without any pain during the past week. The wife emphasizes particularly the long foreplay and the changed attitude, making it possible to gradually replace the old remnants of her upbringing, not in force any more, by new and evident, consistent experiences in her current commitment. But still, the rest of the session was again about religious considerations concerning morals such as self-control, purity, condom prohibition, i.e. sexual arousal without reproduction aims and its supposed "divine legitimacy": "nevertheless it is said, whatever you will bind on earth will also be bound in heaven". By taking these reservations seriously and at the same time calling them into question, a relativization acceptable to the wife could be arrived at and this had the effect of decreasing the distance to the husband's different view. At the end of the session, both emphasized once more that they had "really had a great experience" and now wish to do their best by themselves to keep them going on this path. With that, the therapy ended.

After nearly 2 ½ years the couple returns: "We wanted to give a positive report". They are doing well, living a fulfilling sexuality without any disturbances, she regularly experiences orgasms. Both are particularly impressed by "the general significant increase in life quality and vitality", it is as good as it gets—and the way they present themselves, this seems quite authentic.

This case, closed after only six sessions, concerning what would be called a seemingly anachronistic, religiously induced impairment shows that here again the genuine and effectual causes lie in the frustrated fundamental needs within the partnership. Their primary non-sexual (re-)fulfilment paved the way to a new meaning of sexuality and thus not only eliminated the sexual function disorder, but also achieved a significant increase of general life quality.

The case is typical insofar, as it shows how important it is, not to content oneself with no matter how obvious causes and explanations, without looking underneath for factors on the level of the fundamental needs, which, in the end, ensures durable success and can provide the basis for coping with future problems.

6.5.4   Case Report D

Orgasm Praecox   The chosen passages of the following case history demonstrate very impressively, what a difficult process it can be for patients/couples, to understand and put into action the true objective of the syndyastic focus. In some terms, this process may even make up for lacking "sexual education".

The married couple S. is referred by a psychologist friend (of the therapist). The main complaints are about lacking sexual desire of the wife and the early orgasm of the husband, considering the fact that intercourse is rare and that both have quite different sexual needs. "How is this going to go on?" Both are in their fifties, married for 16 years and have two sons, 14 and 11 years old. Both parents work away from home, he in private industry, she in pharmaceutics. She grew up as an only child (her father did not want children), the parents' marriage was not a happy one, her father was unfaithful to her mother for years. The mother is described as sexually aversive and has taught the daughter that "all men want only the one thing". The wife remembers that—under the pressure of the parental disharmony—she emotionally "shut herself down" at the age of 13. Her desires for tenderness and body contact are small, what the children give her is enough. For years, sexual intercourse took place once a week. "I had to satisfy him. I do not want that any more". Not before a psychotherapy (1 ½ years ago) did she learn to love herself and to "open her heart".

For professional reasons the husband is often away from the family for weeks, has a strong desire for sex, meaning: "satisfaction, affection, tenderness, cuddling". He complains of not enough body contact and closeness to his wife. As a child he had never seen anybody naked and as a result brought an extreme accumulation into his adolescence. Between 11 and 15 years of age he had been at a boys' boarding school, where affection and tenderness were never an issue. At first, his relationships to women were exclusively focused on sex, having "nailed one after the other". Actually, with his wife it was the same. When they were on holidays together, "the hotel room was synonym for sexual intercourse". The conversation revolves around the fundamental needs referred to by the husband and the possibility of their communication and fulfilment through sexuality as an expression of their partnership. The remark made by the therapist of there being many ways of opening oneself immediately affects the wife and she associates "opening the heart" with the opening of genitals. Both seem to have understood, so, as a self-prescribed new experience "caressing (stroking)" as a body language communication method, explicitly excluding coitus is agreed upon and the next session is settled for 1 week later.

In the second session, first the wife reports that she gave in to her husband's pressure of turning caressing (stroking) into foreplay, although she felt resistance and was not sure, whether she/they should? A "huge fury—I am not going to let myself be put under pressure any more" caused a sleepless night. However, the conversation of the last session came to mind. I particularly "remembered understanding that you cannot only open up your heart". Following a mutual talk they successfully undertook a second attempt, both experiencing enjoying closeness, contact and warmth for themselves. After that they went for a walk, but both "floated" more than walked. They felt brand new.

Mr. S.:   It was quite a new experience—I had no idea, I used to take the whole thing as a seduction programme, actually the old programme minus genitals, to get her going, to seduce, because that's what I wanted. But then I realized that it is all about opening to the other, there is more mind concerned and it is very much more affectionate.

Mrs. S.:   You were really there, in the presence, it was wonderful.

Mr. S.:   It was the first time I ever experienced the fact that I didn't even need the sex.

Mrs. S.:   For the first time you really gave me something, it was different than in all the 16 years before, where it was really always about you.

Due to organization reasons the date for the next session was in 3 months time, so it was discussed how these experiences could be repeated and reinforced and explained how the technique of stop/start could be integrated as a control for the climax.

After 3 months the couple returns and makes a happy and liberated harmonious (by no means symbiotic) impression. During the conversation they seem so see things discriminately and sensibly. The man points out the most relevant insights for himself.

Mr. S.:   It always used to be about my dominating drive.

Mrs. S.:   I did not want to be a part of that any more. When he had had his orgasm, nothing else mattered.

Mr. S.:   Up till then, it was all about me, I wanted everything for myself—recently that has changed. I was selfish, the trick is to be able to step back. Since we come here, there is no more masturbation and I am quite able to wait.

Even the orgasm praecox is seen in this context: "To achieve as much as possible in a fast way—that had been a trained program with orgasm as a goal before the partner was able to say no. I was always afraid of the no".

The problem with the orgasm has not been finally solved, but has been diluted within a greater scale. Further training of the stop/start technique is proposed and planned and intensive communication for anxiety reduction aimed at.

For the wife the situation has changed completely. Now, both want to continue.

As a closing remark, Mr. S. points out:

"Conversations such as these should be possible at the age of 20. I am now 55! But there is nothing like that in our society—it should be made compulsory."

6.5.5 Case Report E

Syndyastic Sexual Therapy in a Case of a Paraphilic Arousal Pattern and an Acquired Situational Erectile Disorder Forty-year-old Mr. M. is manager in a small company, confident manner, youthful appearance. For 10 years he has been married to a 6 years younger woman who does part-time administration work at a sports club. Mr. M. is worried and destabilized since 4 weeks ago he was found out in leading a "double life", nearly every week having sexual contact to particularly obese women, weighing 100 kilos and more. This for him incomprehensible inclination has been manifest since his adolescence and there is nothing he can do about it. On the contrary—he has invested much time and effort in organizing according contacts, although he generally had sexual intercourse with each one only once. Only in rare cases did he have sexual contact to one woman more often. After experiencing climax he would find the whole situation disgusting and hate himself for it, particularly with respect to the "infidelity towards my wife", who had, in the meantime, found this out and was totally shocked. His fantasy during masturbation was absorbed to approximately 60 % by these images and he was very worried about the continuation of his marriage. Anyway, he could understand his wife, if she were to divorce him and he had had serious suicidal thoughts. Nevertheless, he was somewhat relieved that his wife knows his secret now, which he had been keeping for 25 years. He loves his wife and wants to try anything to save his marriage.

Going into his sexual biography he reported having had several girlfriends before his marriage, among them also one obese woman, but all these relationships failed, he thinks, because of ever recurring erectile dysfunctions. In fact, these had been a problem from the beginning, also with his present wife of normal weight, who had always coped in a very understanding way with it; this could not, however, prevent chronification. Therefore, 2 years after marriage—even before phosphodiesterase inhibitors were brought onto the market—he learned the handling of auto-injection therapy of the corpora cavernosa and since then was not able to have marital intercourse without it. In the regularly parallel-occurring sexual contacts to obese women, however, he had been capable of erection without auxiliary aids for a considerably long time—but not so in the last years. During sexual intercourse with his wife he also fantasized obese women, which made him feel quite uncomfortable and also like he were cheating on his wife. He presumes that this might be a reason for his reluctant arousal, because he is always trying to suppress the arousing paraphilic images. Indeed, in the light of day, he finds his fantasy images revolting and disgusting. He perceives these obese women as inferior and that is exactly what arouses him. As was revealed later, Mr. M. has had anxieties since childhood about being rejected and with an obese woman these fears are mollified, because with them his feeling is that of complete superiority.

Mrs. M. is a 34-year-old, dark-haired, attractive woman of normal weight with composed conduct, who tries to verbally reconstruct her relationship with suppressed sorrow. Not long after having met her husband, his recurrent erectile dysfunction led to avoidance of intimate contacts, which happened only on her initiative. She put her

husband under pressure to see a urologist for help and agreed to the procedure with
the auto-injection therapy of the corpora cavernosa, because she finds him physically
attractive, wants intimate contact with him and wants to feel his erected penis inside
of her—resulting orgasms were always particularly intensive. Through the auto-
injection treatment their sexual partnership situation had improved, although she
had always experienced him as "tense" during intimate interaction. Now, she was
all the more upset and "deeply disappointed" when she accidentally found a great
amount of contacts to obese women on his computer 4 weeks ago. It was a "real
listing" and all this was completely incomprehensible to her. The loss of trust is
huge, similar to a "landslide". She asks herself if it would ever be possible again to
build up a basis for trust, meaning if he were at all able to be faithful to her. At the
same time, she has the wish to have children with him and start a real family.

During talks about possible goals of therapy, both state the importance of first
of all restoring the basis for trust. He: "It should be like it used to be. . . "; She:
"I would like to trust him again". This was a small start: Since the couple-sessions
here, they would talk to each other more often ("also elsewhere") than they used to and
that they put hope into a therapy procedure that this would continue; they were also
hoping that more intimacy might be possible, in fact right up to sexual intercourse,
which meant a particularly intensive form of physical closeness to her. She explains
that she wants to "feel him inside of her" and he claims how wonderful it is to enter
into her; both confirm that an erection is "obviously" necessary to achieve this and
it is beside the point whether or not this erection comes about through auxiliaries
or not—important is that it comes about relaxed and easily, without anxieties. At
this stage, she relates to his paraphilic inclination of looking for particularly obese
women as a sexual stimulus (called dysmorphophilia) and is worried that he could
have a relapse or that during sexual contact he might not be thinking of her, but of
obese women.

Prior to the beginning of therapy, again it was clearly pointed out that his paraphilic
pattern would not be alterable for a life-time and remain part of his sexual preference
structure—to be understood as completely independent and as having nothing to
do with his affection for her. In his case, it is what is called non-exclusive type of
paraphilia, meaning that next to his sexual interest in her, parallel there is always
the paraphilic stimulus, not of his own choice, feeling burdened by it and really not
wanting to act it out. Vitally important is the aspect of what really connects the two of
them—i.e. their mutual affection—and to revive this for the benefit of both. This is
exactly what the *syndyastic sexual therapy* can achieve. One important requirement
for this is openness and it is a good thing that his inclination is no longer a secret and
that hiding and suppressing have stopped accordingly. Under these circumstances,
they might later be able to react jointly in case the paraphilic impulses gain intensity;
later, additional (e.g. sex-drive suppressing) medication might be an option and this
also has to be decided jointly and supported by her, because it involves reduction
of his sexual impulse dynamics in general. However, the safest protection from any
further disruption of their partnership would be to put it on very stable grounds,
learning to trust and being completely sure and appreciative of one another. On this
basis, it will be possible to realize the non-paraphilic parts of the sexual preference

structure in a non-anxious manner, so that both can mutually enjoy their intimate encounters. This would lead to an increase of partnership and sexual contentedness and considerably reduce the likelihood of a "relapse".

Both partners were able to understand and relate to the concept of the *syndyastic sexual therapy* as a treatment procedure. Already after the first "self-prescribed" new intimate communication they experienced "much more closeness" together, very likely due to her newly found trust in him, because she could feel his openness. At an early stage in therapy, his paraphilic inclination was an issue and he freely provided information. He reports that he inevitably sometimes sees obese women ("after all, they do exist") and that sexual fantasies do pop into his head, but in no way as urgent and intensive as in former times; he ascribes this to the gained transparency and the newly developed trust. He is "no longer alone with it", does "not have to shield things off", does "not need to lie all the time" and this is "extremely relieving".

The following therapy sessions continually showed a mutually appreciative couple, receptive for new experiences. Surprisingly, erectile dysfunctions did not occur any more, either. In his opinion, this was caused by the feeling of complete trust that had developed, by the great closeness to her and the wonderful feeling of security with her.

The conclusive development went quite rapidly. Not only the insertion of the penis but shortly after that the successively agreed upon expansions, stimulating pelvic movements and also being able to reach climax during vaginal penetration (during which he conducted clitoral stimulation) were extremely positive experiences for both partners. Now, more spontaneous, intimate contacts came about, not that they always necessarily lead to sexual intercourse, although he usually had complete erection. Both enjoyed this actively and could indulge in one another, which, from his angle, is worth underlining. Therapeutic interventions were restricted to suggesting getting into intimate situations as openly as possible and not to compare these with past situations and, most of all, to communicate the own emotions. Both were of the opinion that communication on the whole had improved and that this would also reflect itself in intimate communication situations. They are very happy and satisfied with the achieved (see detailed description of therapeutic procedure in this case in Beier and Loewit 2004).

Syndyastic Sexual Therapy and Sexual Preference Viewed superficially, the chosen case example—concerning the path and sequence of the interventions—might leave the impression that the method of this *syndyastic sexual therapy* were nothing enlightingly "new". From the point of view of the experiencing significance and the purpose, however, the focus is on the existentially crucial level of the indispensable psychosocial fundamental needs and thus puts sexuality into a broadened context of meaning. In fact—different from the classic sexual therapy—it is exactly not of any importance to do any "exercises", which should, at the end of therapy, allow previously damaged sexual functions to work again. It is all about mutual fulfilment of fundamental needs (i.e. syndyastic or attachment dimension) for both partners within their relationship, i.e. including their mutual intimacy, in some cases despite impaired sexual function (also see Kleinplatz and Ménard 2007). This is the very reason why, in a disorder of sexual preference or paraphilia, the syndyastic focus is such an appropriate strategy—as long as both partners explicitly want to improve their sexual and partnership contentedness and as long as this can be accomplished by the necessary self-retraction within the partnership. This can only work, if the paraphilic stimulus is subjectively not experienced as being more significant than the attachment itself. This shows at the same time that in diagnostics of paraphilias the exploration of the three dimensions of sexuality (attachment, desire, reproduction) is an indispensable element, because the choice of therapeutic options and the connected chances for development can be assessable.

6.6   Outlook for the Future of (Intimate) Relationships

As far as the future of intimate relationships is concerned, we may definitely, in possession of our knowledge on the evolution of the "socially organized mammal", take for granted that the longing for attachment and relationship will be, as in the past, much stronger and more durable than the varying tides of time. Intimate relationship does, however, need caring for and, if necessary, a helping hand, because the gulf between the longing for a functioning partnership and making it work is widening, following the process of individualization having been promoted by the so-called "post-modern times" of our day and age. Alone the high geographical flexibility taken for granted concerning the place of work may put tight limitations on the taking up, cultivation and continuation of intimate partnerships.

This is where sexual medicine has its preventive task in supporting sexual health and its specific therapeutic task where it is necessary to regain sexual health. In this context, the syndyastic sexual therapy conducts a methodical focus, which is quite different from all other sex therapy approaches: For example, Schnarch (1991, 1997) and also Clement (2004) concentrate on the dimension of sexual desire, most likely meeting the (still undifferentiated) expectations of most patients. All this may be an appealing prospect (and promotional at that), but cannot reach the fundamental variable for the development of desire: the attachment dimension of sexuality.

Indeed, particularly Schnarch, emphasizes its particular significance, but only to—in the long run—regard it as a vehicle to enhance desire. In syndyastic sexual therapy, it is exactly the other way around: The dimension of attachment is therapeutically focused on in the first place, then differentiates the conditions and issues concerning intimacy, as does Schnarch, as well, thus creating a common basis for mutual sexually arousing experiences. This construction is all the more necessary, because for many partners desire and relationship are (at least to begin with) two different realms of experience, connecting gradually during therapy progress and—at its best—evolving into an encompassing experience of lust, when "orgastic" and "attachment" desire blend together.

The widespread dualism or opposition of "sex" and "love" is radically (literally from the roots) revoked by the syndyastic sexological therapy, thus restoring the longed for unity of "desire and attachment".

6.7 Postgraduate Training Programme in Sexual Medicine

In Germany, sexual medicine is accredited in Berlin only (since November 2007) namely as an official postgraduate course according to the standing rules of the Berlin Medical Chamber, but not in other Federal States, showing that this discipline is not adequately integrated into the general medical field yet. However, in Europe there are visible endeavours to improve the situation and in Austria the general accreditation took place in April 2011.

Due to the serious prevalence of sexual disorders and the necessary expertise concerning their assessment and treatment, it would be desirable that appropriate postgraduate education of colleagues in all connected medical disciplines—particularly in gynecology and obstetrics, dermatology and venereology, internal medicine and general medicine, paediatrics, child and adolescent psychiatry, psychiatry and psychotherapy, psychosomatic medicine and urology.

The postgraduate training consists of a theoretical and a practical part, applying an integrative procedure.

Theory The theoretical part covers the acquirement of knowledge concerning evolutionary-biological and socio-cultural basics of human sexuality; anatomical, physiological and psychological (biopsychosocial) basics of sexuality basics of psychosexual and somatosexual development and their process during life span development of gender identity and sexual orientation; sexological relevance of fundamental legal principles (criminal law on sexuality, civil status law, law on transsexuality, medical law, etc.).

The practical clinical part covers the acquisition of knowledge, experience and skills in setting indication and prognostic estimates of psychotherapeutic, somatic and medicational treatment approaches, the identification of psychodynamic and partnership processes of sexuality including conflicts of sexual experience (gender-belonging issues) and behaviour as well as accompanying perceptions and emotions, aetiology, progression and dynamics, diagnostics, classification, prevention, counselling skills and therapy with differentiated indication allocation in disorders of sexual function, sexual development, sexual preference, sexual behaviour, sexual reproduction and gender identity, always also considering them as a consequence of other medical conditions or their treatment or sexual traumatization.

Practice The practical part is based on the acquired knowledge and consists of a 6-months clinical programme to ensure direct contact with patients, which can alternatively be obtained by adequate participation in case conferences at the Department for Sexual Medicine. To achieve certification, a supervision of own sexological assessments and treatment cases in single and couple settings and structured self-experience sessions have to be accounted for.

Chapter 7
New Challenges for Sexual Medicine

7.1 The Internet and the New Media

The impact of the new communication technologies on the psychosexual development of adolescents has not been subject to relevant scientific research yet. In Germany, there are some data available from the "KIM-Study" (2009) stating that 97–99 % of German schools' pupils have internet access and most of these are used on a daily basis or at least on most days a week, making the internet a seriously influential media, without any doubt also in terms of a source for psychosexual experience.

A survey involving 1,228 adolescents between the age of 11 and 17 revealed that 42 % in the 11–13-year-olds and 79 % in the 14–17-year-olds had already viewed sexually explicit (pornographic) images, implying that consumption increases distinctly from 13 years (see results of the "Bravo-Dr.-Sommer-Studie" 2009).

Although there is an obvious gender difference (girls often find pornography disgusting and do not want to see more of it, boys are excited by it and believe to be able to learn from it; cf. Grimm et al. 2010), it is a fact that for the first time in cultural history of man, (not counting singular cases of "forced sex education" by parents in the time of the "68 generation") sexuality is actually learned by viewing images and not, as in the past, by real physical experiences with peers stimulating the educational process.

The easy access to pornographic films—such as via websites like *Youporn* or *Freeporn*—leads to the following situation: Prepubescent minors are able to view sexual interactions, which mostly depict unrealistic forms of sexuality, showing women as objects of sexual interaction, longing for never-ending penetrations and enjoying swallowing great amounts of sperm, best from many different men at the same time. This definitely is not a general feature of common sexual and partnership comfort, which would be a desirable perspective for adolescents (see Chap. 3). However, it would be most naive to assume that these images and films would in no way influence the sexual self-concept and possibly also the sexual preference structure of prepubescent minors (Note: The sexual preference structure, once manifested, is irreversible; see above).

K. M. Beier, K. K. Loewit, *Sexual Medicine in Clinical Practice*,
DOI 10.1007/978-1-4614-4421-3_7, © Springer Science+Business Media, LLC 2013

It has to be assumed that the visually consumed sexual interactions, in self-comparison will be projected in two classifiable characteristics: (see Grimm et al. 2010):

1. Quantitatively: a long penis, large breasts, "good" figure
2. Qualitatively: long-lasting sexual performances, special positions (all of this seemingly effortless).

Even if there is recognition of the fact that such depictions do not represent (average) reality, still they show acts by real people, and are liable to have "exemplary function". The neurobiological basis for this are the mirror neurones, meaning neurones, which trigger the same potentials during image viewing as they would whilst not only (passively) viewing but (actively) acting out these performances. (Their existence was proven recently in humans; see Mukamel et al. 2010).

It is plausible to take for granted that sexual activities are also depicted in the brain by mirror neurones. So, it is to be assumed that things seen by children and adolescents in (pornographic) films lead to a neurophysiological correlation in their brain. This is true in any case, without taking possibly developing sexual preference features into account, and does touch the development of the sexual self-perception and the gender role socialization. The perceived images of sexual performances are automatically judged as an expression of gender-typical behaviour concerning the interaction between men and women. Especially by their (stereotype) repetition, the object character of women is pointedly expressed which leads to a continuation of a subordinate relationship image of male and female, which should have been long since replaced by an image of equal value in both genders, not least because this is an essential precondition for egalitarian intimate relationships.

In addition, it is most troubling to find that by simple online search without any barriers worth mentioning, images of all kinds of paraphilias (including the very seldom ones, see Chap. 4.4) can be found, including illegal images such as sexual violence, sexual contact to animals, acts of child sexual abuse (CSA) etc., which, according to Sabina et al. (2008), at least one-third of a questioned random student sample had seen before the age of 18. It is obvious that this proportion will increase with the rapidly growing improvement of communication technologies. Actually, the attraction of the "taboo breaking" would be a further motivational force to illuminate the darkest corners of these image worlds—to then pass them on via cell phones, be it only to appear "cool" in the eyes of peers.

Although there is no epidemiological data (yet), how this might influence the prevalence of sexual preference disorders of future generations, it is long since known through clinical experience that adolescents in their puberty report on masturbation accompanying fantasies based on pornographic material (pictures or films) previously viewed on the internet. Regularly this concerns youths in need of counselling due to suspicion of preference disorders, for instance when parents have observed that their son preferably consumes images of children in his spare time and have found out about films he has been watching on the internet showing sexual interaction with children.

Based on the idea of a biopsychosocial mixture of factors causing the genesis of sexual preference structure (whether norm-conform or paraphilic), it is justified to assume that, in the case of a possibly existing (nonetheless still unknown) biological predisposition for developing a paraphilia by easy access to paraphilic images, there is practically always a developmental channel.

In reverse, the probability that it would remain "only" a predisposition decreases.

Until proof of the opposite, the general possibility will have to be postulated, that, in children and adolescents, easy access to paraphilic images may lead to an increase of the number of individuals with paraphilic arousal patterns which, in turn, would lead to effects on relationships and partnership contentedness (see above).

A recent survey of a group of (Croatian) students showed that (regular) users of paraphilic images (compared with users of non-paraphilic internet pornography) consume pornography at an earlier age and more intensively, have a higher masturbation frequency, experience more sexual boredom, are more orientated on myths concerning sexuality, show greater sexual impulsiveness and experience less intimacy and sexual comfort (see Stulhofer et al. 2010).

This would also apply to the influence on the frequency of sexual function disorders. Even now it can be stated that hypoactive sexual desire and orgasm disorders in women have been attributed to—at that time (e.g. at the age of 17) found disgusting—pornography films. Although currently involved in a loving partnership, at that time, sexuality was negatively stigmatised and separated from love. In any assessment of young adults, the direct question concerning pornography exposition or, to the point, the starting age of viewing such pictures or films and their influence on the personally experienced significance of sexuality must never be left out.

7.1.1 *"Cyber Bullying" and "Online Grooming"*

For prepubescent and pubescent minors, the internet and the new communication technologies are by no means virtual spaces, detached from their own reality—rather they serve as an integral component of their every-day life in which they communicate, display themselves (image cultivation), seek information, etc. Here they are not only confronted (more or less inadvertently) with pornographic, but also with violent and harmful contents.

An always increasing status is becoming ever popular by deliberately causing damage to others in the sense of bullying, hassling, insulting, blackmailing, excluding and sexual harassing through the use of the new media (see McCabe and Martin 2005; Lösel and Bliesener 2003).

This phenomenon is also described as "cyber bullying" and is a special form of mobbing to be taken very seriously (see Menesini and Nocentini 2009). For example, via mobile phone text, photo- or video-threats, insults, harassments are sent or malicious gossip or harmful made-up stories—sometimes without the knowledge of the person concerned—are spread mainly to peers.

In "mobile bullying", there is no given security barrier whatsoever, because the malicious messages are sent via mobile phones and there is no stopping them being passed on further and thus spreading without control. For the concerned victims, the situation gets worse, if, for example embarrassing photographs or videos, which are intended to exclude this person, come to the attention of a more or less large circle of fellow pupils. In an early study by Lösel and Bliesener (2003), they had been able to show that bullying victims are characterized by problems such as anxiety, depressive moods, social withdrawal and psychosomatic complaints, which points out the vulnerability of adolescents for these kinds of attacks.

As far as the offenders are concerned, certain familial risks (lacking emotional warmth, aggressive upbringing, instable norm orientation), personality factors (impulsiveness, little self-control, lacking of competent social information processing), particularities of the peer group (aggressive dissociation toward other groups) and a preference for violent media contents seem to play a role (see Lösel and Bliesener 2003).

The results of the survey by Grimm and Rhein (2007) show clearly that the effects, such as social stigmatization and social isolation caused by these modern forms of mobbing can be very serious indeed.

By now, the percentage of adolescents having become victims of cyber bullying, is estimated at 20–40 %, whereas neither age nor gender can count as predictors, but inevitably serious psychosocial, emotional and school-related problems arise (Tokunaga 2009).

According to a study by Calvete et al. (2010), 44 % of the questioned had been actively involved in "cyber bullying"—boys more than girls. This behaviour was prevalent, when the offenders, to a greater extent, had had experiences with violence as well as a disposition for aggressive behaviour and were not generally relying on social support from friends.

The high prevalances, both in the case of victims as in offenders, make clear that here a serious problem for adolescent development in general has arisen, which has to be reckoned with on top of the other influences of the new media mentioned above.

In this context, it is necessary to mention the counterpart of "cyber bullying", the (alleged) caring "grooming" in social networks, in which by friendly attention (at least at first) trust is built up, in order for instance to acquire photos of the victims or even a personal meeting, which, again, may result in sexual traumatization, due to the fact that often the committers are not young people at all. They are adults, who, possibly acting on their own sexual interests (namely due to a pedophilic or a hebephilic inclination; see Chaps. 4.4 and 7.2) try to contact adolescents or children via the social networks, stating a wrong, much younger age, pretending to be somebody else, for instance a peer wanting to become a new friend.

In a study by Shannon (2008), evaluating data of the Swedish Law Enforcement Authorities on "Online Sexual Grooming", 87 % of the offenders were more than 18 years of age and 71 % of the victims less than 14 years old.

Wolak et al. (2007) have worked out nine items, marking these as risky internet behaviour: (1) posting personal information online; (2) interacting online with people not known in person; (3) having unknown people on a buddy list; (4) using the internet to make rude and nasty comments to others; (5) sending personal information to unknown people met online; (6) downloading images from file-sharing programmes; (7) visiting X-rated sites on purpose; (8) using the internet to embarrass or harass people youths are mad at; and (9) chatting online to unknown people about sex.

During their own survey, Wolak et al. (2007) found out that three quarters of internet users between the age of 10 and 17 own up to at least one of these risky behaviours, nearly one-third had stated having even 4 (and more).

According to Mitchell et al. (2001), the following "criteria" are connected to an especially high risk of becoming a victim of sexual harassment: female gender, aged between 14 and 17, dealing with psychological conflicts, high-frequency use of the internet, preferably in chat rooms, communicating with strangers.

In contrast, knowledge concerning committer behaviour is confined to certain individual case analyses (see Marcum 2007) which do, however, show impressively, with how much manipulative communication skills committers proceed in their aim to involve the victims in issues of sexual content.

All this shows the necessity of improved framework conditions for preventive measures (in media education as well) ascribing parents but also social workers and teachers an important part in this vital process.

7.2 Primary Prevention of Child Sexual Abuse (CSA) and the Use of Child Abusing Images (CP)

Men with pedophilia are responsible for 40 % of CSA (see Beier 1998; Seto 2008). Pedophilia is defined as the erotic preference for the body scheme of prepubescent children, which can determine sexual orientation of the inclined individual either completely (exclusive type) or partly (non-exclusive type) (see APA 2000).

As sexual preference structure is established during adolescence and from then on manifest for a life-time, i.e. *unconvertible*, this also applies to any occurring particularities of preference structure such as pedophilia (see Chap. 4.4). For men with this pedophilic inclination it means that since puberty they have been living with sexual arousal fantasies about children's bodies and that they have had to control these impulses, in order not to become an offender and not to traumatize children, not even on the internet by using child-abusing images.

It needs to be clearly stated that no-one can "choose" their sexual preference structure, it is "fate and not choice", which is why it would be amiss to condemn this by moral standards, only—and then quite rightly—if sexual fantasies are *acted out* and impair others (in the case of pedophilia meaning children) in their individuality and integrity (see Chap. 4.5).

The other 60 % of CSA cases are not based on sexual preference disorders of the offenders in the sense of pedophilia. The offences take place as the so-called "substitute acts" with surrogate partners, substituting sexual interaction with a preferred adult partner, which—for whatever reason, e.g. due to personality disorder or mental retardation—cannot be adequately socially achieved (see Chap. 4.5).

Nevertheless, in the case of sexual preference for minors, an increased risk level for repeated CSA has to be anticipated (see Hanson and Morton-Bourgon 2005). Therefore, recidivism rates in pedophilic preference offenders lie between 50 and 80 %, while in otherwise motivated offenders it was 10–30 % (see Beier 1998). In addition to that, a pedophilic inclination predestinates the use of child-abusive images (belittlingly called "child pornography"), because pedophiles are sexually particularly drawn to images of children and are therefore at increased risk to regularly view, download and collect child-abusive images (see Seto et al. 2006). It is also a fact that in the majority of the "hands-on" abuse offences of children and the use of child-abusive images there are no charges filed, no lawful prosecution and no registration by the justice system. This is the so-called *Dunkelfeld* (literally meaning "dark field"; see Pereda et al. 2009).

This connection between sexual preference and sexual behaviour is all the more alarming when considering the first epidemiological data revealing that prevalence of pedophilic inclination is approximately 1 % of the male population (in women it is a rarity; see Ahlers et al. 2009). By way of illustration: These figures coincide with the prevalence of Parkinson's disease and justify an estimate of 250,000 individuals concerned in Germany.

Pedophilic men are therefore to be considered *the most important target-group of primary prevention* of CSA and of "consumption of child-abusive images" in the Dunkelfeld.

Besides pedophilia, there is another paraphilia called hebephilia, i.e. sexual attraction towards early pubescent body scheme (development stage with beginning growth of pubic hairs and breasts, i.e. Tanner stages 2 and 3—not to be confused with ephebephilia or parthenophilia; see Chap. 4.4). It is an independent disorder of sexual preference to be diagnosed according to the International Classification System of the World Health Organization (ICD-10) or the American Psychiatric Association (DSM-IV-TR), not yet specifically coded (for DSM-V there are plans to change this; see Blanchard et al. 2008). However, it must be kept in mind that in industrial countries, the onset of puberty is averagely around the age of 11 for both genders.

The "Prevention Project Dunkelfeld" A primary prevention therapy programme dealing with pedophilically and hebephilically inclined men at the risk for sexual offending against children but until then not having acted upon their impulses and dealing with real offenders at risk to re-offend in the *Dunkelfeld* (which is a secondary preventive approach) was established in June 2005 in Germany (and therefore first worldwide) under the research project "Prevention of CSA in the *Dunkelfeld*" at the *Institute for Sexology and Sexual Medicine* at the University Clinic Charité in Berlin. At the beginning, the project was financially supported by the *Volkswagen Foundation* and since 2008 also—due to special commitment of the Ministry for Justice—state aided by government funds. It is also supported by the Child Protection Organization *Foundation Hänsel + Gretel* as well as by the international media agency *scholz and friends*.

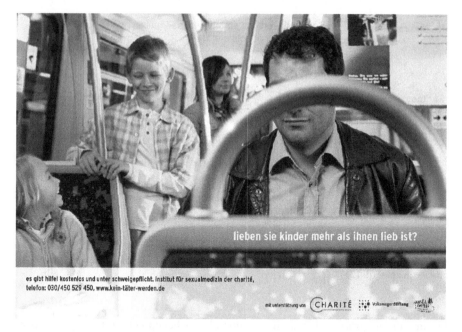

es gibt hilfe! kostenlos und unter schweigepflicht. institut für sexualmedizin der charité,
telefon: 030/450 529 450, www.kein-täter-werden.de

mit unterstützung von (CHARITÉ ⁝•⁝ Volkswagenstiftung ⁝ANNELA⁝

Fig. 7.1 Billboard for the media campaign "Dunkelfeld", drafted by Scholz and friends. Meaning: "Do you like children in ways you shouldn't? Don't offend. There is help—free of charge and confidential." (p. 125)

Self-motivated men fitting the target group were successfully alerted by a media campaign about the opportunity to join the prevention project, *free of charge* and protected by the pledge of *medical confidentiality,* and thus obtain diagnostic expertise as well as qualified consultation, i.e. therapy offers (Fig. 7.1).

Basically, the offered therapy consists of three blocks as an expression of a biopsychosocially based treatment: *Sexological intervention* promotes self-acceptance of the sexual preference and its integration into the self-concept and is aimed at involvement of relatives or partners in the therapeutic process; *cognitive behaviour therapy methods* improve self-regulation strategies of the pedophiles concerning a general changing attitude towards sexuality, capability of perspective responsibility, successful emotion-coping and stress-handling as well as conflict management within a partnership; with the help of *pharmacotherapy* (serotonin re-uptake inhibitors; anti-androgene medication such as Cyproteronacetat or GnRH-Analoga) sexual impulses can additionally be modulated and thus effectively reduce offence risk (Fig. 7.2)

By February 2010, 1,134 men had responded; 499 of them had fully completed diagnosis and 255 had been offered a therapy place. These men came from mixed social backgrounds, had averagely known about their sexual inclination since the age of 22, and averagely joined the project at the age of 39. More than half had previously tried for therapeutic help elsewhere without success. Total 48 % of the interview partners had travelled more than 100 km to take part in the study. It turned

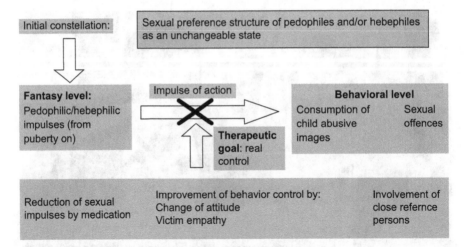

Fig. 7.2 Sexological intervention model for the prevention of CSA and the consumption of child-abusive images. (p. 126)

out that the majority had, indeed, a pedophilic or hebephilic preference disorder, and many of these men additionally showed emotional stress symptoms (especially depression and anxiety) which can be evaluated as an expression of the often-existing comorbidity (see Beier et al. 2009).

The Prevention Project Child-Abusive Images Supported by the Federal Ministry of Family Affairs, in 2009, an expansion of the prevention offers for potential and real offenders (not known to the justice system) took place, in this case with focus on potential and undetected real users of child-abusive images. It was based on knowledge from the Prevention Project Dunkelfeld stating, that half the number of potential offenders were already users of child-abusive images showing very low sense of guilt (see Beier and Neutze 2009). Further analysis of this group revealed a connection between age and activity: The youngest group had neither used child-abusive images nor had they abused a child "hands on". With increasing age of the participants, the probability increased that one of these offenses (or both) had been done. This suggests to try reaching pedophilic men before they start using child-abusive images, for which they are predestinated by their preference disorder. Regarding this, a TV spot and an internet banner was produced in order to reach the target group of users in the web. It is a fact that in many cases, pedophiles are not socially isolated, but are integrated into social networks, have a family or a partnership. Therefore, the new project is also aimed at general information for the public concerning "consumption of child-abusive images" and the exceptional situation for users who—due to their (pedophilic/hebephilic) preference disorder—need to withstand the temptation of using these images, saving, downloading, collecting or exchanging them.

Outlook The gathered experiences from the Prevention Project of the Berlin Charité has been able to show that in the Dunkelfeld it is possible to actually prevent—if not everyone, nevertheless a great many—CSA and child pornography offenses, where in the past nothing was done at all.

Therapeutic prevention offers are taken on by self-motivated pedophiles and hebephiles, if they themselves want to prevent CSA or consumption of child-abusive images for the first time (potential offenders) or any repetition (in real Dunkelfeld offenders). Nevertheless, due to the inconvertibility of the pedophile preference structure, it is a chronic disease and therefore a life-long general problem to be dealt with, so, to enable useful prevention work, an accessible "chronic disease management programme" needs to be established, not only in Berlin but in other German states and other countries as well. It has to be emphasized that the required facilities will only reach the target group on a primary preventive level if established outside of a psychiatric or even forensic context. In any case, the whole spectrum of specific medically indicated therapy offers (including pharmaceutical options to modulate sexual impulses) need to be made available.

7.3 Sexual Traumatization and Therapeutic Approaches for Victims

7.3.1 Epidemiology

The findings by Wetzels (1997) show, within the general German population, a prevalence of sexual abuse experience *prior to the age of 16* in women ranging from 8.6 (hands-on offenses) to 13.8 % (including hands-off offenses) and in men from 2.8 to 4.3 %. These figures roughly reflect the known victim proportion of 75 % female and 25 % male children (see Beier 1995). In international comparison of retrospective representative population studies, the figures for Germany are still at quite a low level (Finkelhor 1994; Pereda et al. 2009). For estimation of the annual incidence in Germany, only the criminal police statistics are available. In this context, it is always emphasized that in offences of CSA, the cover-up efforts of the offenders and the speechlessness and the helplessness of the victims, make it very likely that only a fraction of the offences that have actually taken place are ever uncovered.

For Germany, there are approximately 15,000 cases annually registered in the criminal police statistics. These figures refer to reported cases, the so-called "Hellfeld", which, again according to criminal prosecution statistics, lead in only one-fifth to prosecution of an offender. As far as the extent of the "Dunkelfeld" is concerned, i.e. sexual traumatization not registered by the justice system, only estimations can be made (see Beier et al. 2005).

The prevalence of sexual traumatization *after the age of 16*, at least in women, has been estimated by a representative study of the German Ministry for Family Affairs (BMFSFJ 2004) involving 10,264 women between the age of 16 and 85 years and has

Table 7.1 Short-term behavioural problems and hints relating to child sexual abuse

Non-specific	Highly Suspicious	Specific
Age-dependent	"Sexualized behaviour in	Not known
Vague abdominal pain without	childhood" cave: normal	
morphological correlate	knowledge on sexuality and	
Eating disorders	sexual behaviour at childhood	
Sleeping disorders	age not manifest!	
Fear of abandonment and attacks of		
clinging, but also rejection of contact,		
behavioural regression (bed-wetting,		
encopresis)		
Concentration disorders		
Worsening school results		
Behavioural disorders with varying		
degrees of severity; in boys more		
external, i.e. (sexually) aggressive up		
to delinquent, subversive; in girls		
more internalized (depressed,		
submissive up to suicidal attempts)		
Depression		

generally been confirmed by data from other industrial countries. According to this study, 37 % of the questioned women had, since the age of 16, experienced physical violence and 13 % had actually been victims of sexual abuse. The last-mentioned category included rape (6 %), attempted rape (4 %), violent physical coercion to non-consenting sexual acts (8 %) and coercion to look at pornographic material (1 %). Total 25 % of all women reported to have been physically and/or sexually abused by their (previous or current) partners and 58 % of the questioned women reported on having had some sort of sexual abuse experience in a broader sense in their lives.

7.3.2 Short-Term Consequences

Regarding short-term consequences of sexual abuse and its provable symptoms in children, Beitchmann (1991) and Kendall-Tackett (1997) both come to the conclusion that there are—except the so-called "sexualized behaviour" during childhood, which is extremely difficult to validate—no specific behavioural clues which indicate sexual abuse having taken place. Fundamentally, it can only be noted that children react to sexual abuse with the same unspecific behavioural conspicuousness arising as a reaction to other psychological trauma (Table 7.1).

Using any misinterpretation of such behaviour as "proof" for abuse having taken place without taking other particularities of the child into account, its specific individual mode of expression, its family context and other particularities of its personal surroundings, etc. is liable to cause as much damage as failing to recognize an abuse would.

Table 7.2 Morphological references of child sexual abuse

Non-specific	Highly suspicious	Specific
Hematomas, strangulation marks, fissures, scratch marks (recurrent), inflammation in the anogenital region	Sexually transmitted diseases Hymenal defects	Evidence of sperm (fluids)

This has been demonstrated painfully in many spectacular trials, in which families have been disrupted and children have been traumatized due to unfounded accusations and obsessive exaggerations of random symptoms by self-appointed "helpers and experts" (see Rutschky and Wolff 1994). Consequently, according to all existing data, it can be stated that there is no such thing as a specific "post-sexual-abuse-syndrome"!

No less difficult to determine—because equally unspecific—is the medical provability of physical abuse effects (see Table 7.2). Particularly, seeing that the not seldomly discussed hymen findings are (with sometimes postulated "specific damages", etc.), taking into account the extreme variability of healthy and all the more pathologically altered hymen, only to be judged and interpreted by forensically very-experienced child gynecologists and only in context with other findings derived from the social behavioural context.

7.3.3 Long-Term Consequences

Even more difficult than the evaluation of short-term consequences and short-term symptoms of CSA seems to be the categorization and evaluation of long-term consequences. This can be put down to the fact that unimpaired as well as impaired mental state and behaviour are always the result of a highly complex, interactional and multifunctional ("biopsychosocial") cause context and that they are not reducible to one single factor alone. In fact, various studies have shown that there is no defined late syndrome of CSA and that the markedness of various long-term consequences always depends on both negatively cumulating and protective factors. Of course, meta-analytic studies can only deliver an overall summary. In therapeutic work, it is always about evaluation of *each individual case*. However, on the grounds of the available studies, it can be said that the following factors are likely to generally increase the risk of negative, usually dynamic long-term effects. This means that the traumatization incident and the personal proximity to the perpetrator have effects on the long-term consequences. For example: Being confronted by an exhibitionist just once definitely does not lead to long-term consequences for the child. It can even come to terms with an incident of indecent fondling or one single massive abuse by a stranger without grave consequences, if this child is growing up in a sheltered, caring and trusting family atmosphere, where it receives support and advice and the incident is not unnecessarily dramatized. This protective effect within family atmosphere ("buffering effect") to overcome trauma consequences has always been an issue in developmental psychology (see Kinzl 1997).

It is exactly the lack of this protective effect in the so-called "abuse families" which causes the psycho-toxic factor for the repeatedly described massive psychiatrically relevant long-term consequences in victims of intra familiar abuse. This conduct, usually going on for years and characterized by massive (penetrative) acts of abuse, is done by one person, exactly that person who originally ought to be the one supplying trust and shelter, the one who should help build up the "sense of basic trust". In addition, this isolated inner familiar situation leads to a circle of influence from which the child cannot escape and which puts it at the mercy of the offender. The perpetrators of intra familiar abuse are very often capable of preventing exposure by subtle threats ("If you tell, something will happen to you!"), by strategies of corruption ("You are my very favourite!"), accusations causing feelings of guilt ("Come on, you wanted it, too, we both did it!") and appealing to family solidarity ("If you tell, I will go to prison and you will go to a foster home!"). Quite often, very much later, for instance when victims are grown up and are not living at home anymore and/or are involved in a partnership of their own, it comes to disclosure of having been abused. Sometimes it is because of wanting to spare a younger sibling of also being abused. Other than often claimed, intra familiar CSA is not an ubiquitous phenomenon to be found in all levels of society, rather it happens more often in socially marginal, isolated families. In addition, these are often characterized by non-sexual violence against children and partners, not seldom (!) enhanced by alcohol abuse and without social safeguards (Wetzels 1997)—factors multiplying each other, so that it is retrospectively impossible to later relate the shown symptoms and behavioural abnormalities in the victims solely to CSA. Ultimately, it is all about the sense of basic trust, self-confidence and self-determination, actually a toxic blend of negative developmental conditions. As a consequence of such abuse-triggering multiple constellations (i.e. not only, but definitely also, the sexual abuse), in grown-ups there are often:

Increased depression rate (up to auto-aggression and suicide).
Increased rates of panic disorders and anxiety syndromes.
Increased rate of substance abuse.
Low rates in feelings of self-value and self-confidence.
Increased risk for re-victimisation (i.e. a woman who, as a child, had been sexu-
    ally intra-familiarly abused over a longer time period, has an increased risk of
    becoming a rape victim).

These symptoms (similar to their societal factors as well) occur in different combinations (see Table 7.3).

Effects of Child Sexual Abuse on Sexuality   Looking at the massive infringement—particularly in the course of intra-familiar sexual abuse occurring over a longer period of time—on the sexual autonomy and consequently the impaired manifestation of any originary trust or self-confidence, taking into account the massive humiliation to which the victim is constantly exposed to, the allocation of the sexual domain to fear, pain, shame and feelings of guilt, it seems quite expectable that the sexual

Table 7.3 Variables concerning the development of long-term consequences of experienced child sexual abuse in adults

Problems	Meaningful factors	Tendencies found
Definition	Duration of abuse (once vs. continually)	Sexual function disorders
Age limit	Relationship/closeness to offender (stranger vs.	Re-victimization
Retrospection	family member)	Homosexual experiences
Samples	Severity of abuse (penetration vs. exhibition-	Gender identity disorders
Control groups	ism)	Anxiety disorders
	Use of/threatening of violence	Depressions
	Communication opportunities (particularly the	Suicidal thoughts
	role of the mother)	Suicide attempts
	Procedure of investigation authorities	Drug use/prostitution

experiencing ability and relationship skills of the individuals concerned in their adult lives would be gravely disturbed, if not completely destroyed.

At the same time, epidemiological studies show (see Mullen 1997) that a general existence of classifiable restrictions in sexual function, experience and attachment ability in adults with a history of sexual abuse cannot automatically be taken for granted. There are, however, next to a number of different disorder processes, such as early uptake of promiscuitive sexual relationships (not seldom an expression of the search for comfort and security in adolescents, who know human relationships only in sexualized forms) sexual function disorders in different extents, sexually delinquent behaviour (only in men), some inconspicuous long-term processes with no impaired sexual experiencing in stable relationships (see Leitenberg et al. 1989; Rind et al. 1998). Positive outcomes could be related to the following facts:

- Human development processes are extremely pliable: A victim once does not mean always a victim!
- Present studies have possibly not differentiated enough between individual factors within the abuse process and beyond that within the specific social structure in each separate case. In fact, consequences of sexual abuse are not only dependent on its duration and intensity, but also on protective (familial) factors.
- Very few examiners differentiate specific disorders of sexual experience and behaviour (such as according to DSM-IV-TR).
- It appears that there are gender-typical impact outcomes for later sexual impairments caused by previous CSA, whereas sufficient long-term data is lacking, particularly for male victims.
- Ultimately, sufficient representative data on the prevalence of different sexual disorders within the general population is missing, so that there is no way of stating, whether a certain disorder rate of an abused population is higher, lower or equal in comparison to the not abused population.

Detection of Abuse Experiences as a Cause for Sexual Disorders   On the other hand, in clinical (non-epidemiological) studies as well as in every-day clinical practice, there are repeated indications of abuse experience in patients with sexual function disorder(s).

Many patients have concealed such experiences for reasons of shame, so that individual consultation should cautiously approach this issue, e.g. by asking the question whether the patient has had many sexual experiences in his life (explicitly relating to childhood—many patients regard that part of their life as the "non-sexual part"!) which were uncomfortable or embarrassing, about which he/she has never spoken to anyone before, which happened against his/her will but perhaps with some sort of agreement on his/her part. If questions similar to this are answered in the affirmative, it is necessary to cautiously follow-up, whether it was a one-off experience or if it went on for a duration of time and whether he/she had ever shared this with others (particularly his/her partner). Subsequently, details concerning persons involved, nature and extent of incidents, use of physical violence or verbal threats, etc. should be sensitively extracted (see the additionally influencing factors mentioned above).

Should this line of questioning (not necessarily restricted to 1 hour) lead to the recognition that the patient had been a victim of sexual abuse during childhood, it is necessary to keep in mind:

- That the whole constellation of the traumatizing factors keep on affecting the individual during adulthood and
- That unilinear, monocausal disorder explanations are not useful.

Clearly, a one-off sexual incident with a stranger is not an appropriate explanation for the condition suffered from, compared with a continuously repeated penetrative abuse by a family member. It must therefore be estimated, whether or not the patient is in need of skilled sexological and psychotherapeutic treatment, because, behind the initially claimed sexual disorder symptoms there might be further deeper lying mental disorders hidden. This can particularly be the case in long-term intra-familiar abuse history.

7.3.4 Treatment

For children and adolescents, the experience of sexual abuse may make trauma-therapeutical intervention necessary. Irrespective of the kind of trauma and the post-trauma disorders (see above), as well as the identifiable co-morbidity disorders, it is always crucial that treatment takes into account the developmental psychopathological perspective, meaning giving attention to the developmental age of the concerned individual (see Landolt 2010).

The following treatment options are available:

- Trauma-centred cognitive-behavioural therapy (individual or group settings).
- Trauma-centred psychodynamic play therapy.
- Narrative exposition therapy for children.
- EMDR (eye movement and desensitization processing therapy).
- Psychodynamic, hypnotherapeutic, family-therapeutic and systemic-orientated methods.
- The administration of medication (pharmacotherapy).

Discussion of Current Procedures The clearest evidence is based on results from trauma-centred cognitive-behavioural therapies, but also the EMDR and the narrative exposition therapy with children come up with high evidence scores (see Landolt 2010). As far as all other methods are concerned, there are only evidence scores of clinical effectiveness so that strict scientific proof of any benefit is still pending. It has to be stated, however, that even for the methods with high-efficacy scores not all data concerning the treatment of children who have experienced sexual abuse are available—with the exception of the trauma-focused cognitive behavioural therapy, for which, in turn there are meta-analytical studies at hand (see Amand et al. 2008). These came to the remarkable conclusion that obviously a decisive efficacy factor seems to be precisely the influencing of parents and close persons, meaning that their involvement must be of important value. Naturally, all this leads to a number of implications, ultimately concerning the case management from the first day on, because there is a huge difference whether there are attempts to involve the social system (in fact systematically, as is the case within the cognitive-behavioural therapy programme) or, on the contrary, aiming at separation from persons of the close social network, in particular when intra-family abuse is suspected. Anyway, the effects of evaluated therapy programmes indicate that it is wise to strengthen the inner familial position of the child by therapy, thus making use of exactly that "buffer effect", which seems to represent the crucial curative factor: Just the fulfilment of the fundamental needs for acceptance, appreciation, security and safety supplied by the closest attachment persons.

If the symptoms are limited to a sexual function disorder (difficult to diagnose), generally the same principles for treatment apply, as described in Chaps. 5 and 6. The communication-orientated understanding of human sexuality calls for a certain approach: The patient's experienced abuse, and particularly if it had been kept from the partner, needs to be included within the couple-centred therapy. It is the only way for both partners to deal with the partnership-impairing trauma or even, ideally, to overcome this trauma experience completely (see Nijs 1997). In the course of this, it might be helpful to explain to both that the "buffer function", which might have failed to work in the victim's primary family, can now be taken on by both partners and that this would help to heal the wounds of the soul. The aim should be, not to give the offender any "power" at all over his previous victim, allowing him—quasi from a distance or retrospectively—to further compromise his/her ability of experience.

Case Report 16 A 25-year-old man with a history of multiple sexual traumatizations at the age of 10.

The patient, at first impression quiet and thoughtful but lacking emotion, worked as a storekeeper and had been in a relationship with a 3 years younger woman, whom he described as the "woman of my life" and with whom he wanted to start a family. Progressively worrying was a generalized orgasm disorder, which arose during sexual intercourse as well as during masturbation. The patient reported as to having no sexual fantasies at all during masturbation and to concentrate completely on his girlfriend during sex, but at the same time of being disappointed each time when he did not reach climax. Only at night, during sleep did he have ejaculations.

Further assessment revealed a series of abuse incidents for more than a period of approximately 1 year by the stepfather, whom the mother was economically dependent upon and who terrorized the whole family at that time (the patient had a 5 years younger brother). At the time of the abuse, he had been 10 years old and had then been sent to a foster home for bad behaviour—he believes that this way his mother wanted to put an end to the abuse by the stepfather, but they had never spoken about this to each other. At the age of 15, he had confided in a care worker, it came to criminal charges, later to court procedures ending with conviction and a prison sentence of several years for the perpetrator. He had had to give evidence at the trial. Usually, the stepfather had demanded of him to stimulate him manually or orally and in case of refusal he would threaten that he (the stepfather) would leave the family and not support them anymore. (The accuracy of his evidence was confirmed by the verdict, of which he had brought a written copy to the next therapy session.) A therapeutic processing of this traumatization had never taken place. In the context of the sexological intervention it was attempted to unburden him with regard to the experiences and to offer him the unique opportunity of seeing the relationship to his girlfriend as a chance to fulfil the frustrated psychosocial fundamental needs (for acceptance, security, etc.) and thus to stabilize the syndyastic function level, which would be a precondition for an appreciative integration of the body and the genitals in terms of intimate contact to a beloved person. In the duration of the treatment, the patient started developing fantasies (gynephile orientation, vaginal-penetrative practices), was able to accept these during masturbation, i.e. allow himself to use stimulating pornographic material and in a first step reach orgasm during masturbation, later on also during coital intimacy, this still being easily susceptible to interference. Increasingly, he was able to build up trust in the success of the relationship, because he felt he was authentically being wanted and loved and not utilized. The greater problem was caused by the fact that his mother still vehemently refused to deal with that particular phase of their family life and left it at comments about her husband having been a "bad person"—leaving her own personal involvement concerning her inability of keeping her children safe out of the issue.

The Central Role of the Dimension of Attachment   Early traumatic life experiences are remarkably common and can—according to results from epidemiological studies—have far-reaching, harmful consequences on mental and physical health of an individual, even decades later (see Flaherty et al. 2009 with results of the "Adverse Childhood Experiences" ACE-Study, with 17,421 adult participants in the USA). Neurobiological research is more and more convinced that traces of early childhood traumatization can be detected in the brain itself and can influence brain volume of various structures (such as the hippocampus) or the activation pattern of different brain regions (see Gündel and Stephan 2010). As neuronal networks, the hypothalamus–hypophysal–gonadal axis, as well as the sympathical nerve system play an important role with corresponding discharge of hormones or catecholamines, which not only control the vegetative excitability, but also directly the immune system (see Bauer 2005). Furthermore, messenger substances such as cytokines are released, but, in fact also neuropeptides such as oxytocin, which is known for its ability of stabilizing psycho-emotional feelings such as trust, security and safety by relieving anxiety and reducing the activation of the amygdala (see, e.g. Kirsch et al. 2005) or also by increasing the ability of empathy for others (see Domes et al. 2007).

Thus, it is not surprising that a linkage has been found between childhood traumatization and low(er) oxytocin levels in the spinal fluid of afflicted persons (Heim et al. 2009). This corresponds with the outcome of a study involving undergraduate students concerning their willingness to charitable donating after oxytocin administration: The positive effect of oxytocin administration on pro-social behaviour was moderated by experiences of parental love withdrawal, i.e. it seems limited to individuals with supportive backgrounds (Ijtzendoorn et al. 2011).

The alleged connections between the above-mentioned systems are shown in Fig. 6.1 (see Chap. 6), illustrating how closely oxytocin is linked to the "syndyastic system", looking at it as a particular feature of the "social brain" and consequently how strongly future research should go into neurohormonal basics of attachment ability in order to obtain an improved understanding of the connection between early childhood traumatization and mental and physical disease in adults in order to widen the possibilities of early detection and specific therapeutic intervention (see Gündel and Stephan 2010). Without doubt, this will be a task for the whole of society (see Shonkoff 2009).

It also displays that it is exactly the frustration of human fundamental needs for trust, security and safety in the experience of child sexual abuse that may represent the main traumatizing influence factor, which is all the more serious, if it is present in other spheres of the life of the child or adolescent, meaning there is nowhere to turn for the necessary appreciation, acceptance and security at all for the victim. Furthermore, it is obvious that in biopsychosocial understanding, attachment is a definite constituent of sexuality and needs special attention: First, it is present in body language and then also in verbal communication (verbalizing the emotions) with reliable close persons. Therefore, sexuality is a particularly intensive way of letting body language communication create, express and deepen attachment between individuals. To uncover these correlations and to experience their meaning in the so-called self-agreed-upon "new experiences" (see Chap. 6.3), conveys a new dimension of sexuality, which has nothing whatsoever to do with the past traumatizing incident(s) and is not at all comparable, even if superficially it might appear to be the same. This means that the dimension of attachment (or syndyastic dimension of sexuality) and its applicable syndyastic sexual therapy may change attachment deficits in a healing sense—even after (sexual) traumatization—and help increase life quality and well-being.

References

Ahlers, C. J., Schaefer, G. A., & Beier, K. M. (2005). Das Spektrum der Sexualstörungen und ihre Klassifizierbarkeit im ICD-10 und DSM-IV. *Sexuologie, 12,* 120–152.

Ahlers, C. J., Schaefer, G. A., Mundt, I. A., et al. (2011). How unusual are the contents of paraphilias—prevalence of paraphilia-associated sexual arousal patterns (PASAPs) in a community-based sample of men. *Journal of Sexual Medicine, 8,* 1362–1370.

Althof, S. E. (2006). Prevalence, characteristics and implications of premature ejaculation/rapid ejaculation. *Journal of Urology, 175,* 842–848.

APA. (American Psychiatric Association) (2000). *Diagnostic and statistical manual of mental disorders fourth edition revised (DSM-IV-TR).* Washington: APA-Press.

Balint, M. (1965). Die Urformen der Liebe und die Technik der Psychoanalyse. Bern/Stuttgart: Huber, Klett.

Balint M. (1957). Der Arzt, sein Patient und die Krankheit. Klett, Stuttgart.

Bartels, A., & Zeki, S. (2004). The neural correlates of maternal and romantic love. *NeuroImage, 21*(3), 1155–1166.

Basson, R. (2000). The female sexual response: A different model. *Journal of Sex and Marital Therapy, 26,* 51–65.

Basson, R. (2002). Neubewertung der weiblichen sexuellen Reaktion. *Sexuologie, 9*(1), 23–29.

Bauer, M. E. (2005). Stress, glucocorticoids and ageing of the immune system. *Stress, 8,* 69–83.

Becker, S., Bosinski, H. A. G., Clement, U., et al. (1997). Standards der Behandlung und Begutachtung von Transsexuellen. *Sexuologie, 4,* 130–138.

Beier, K. M. (1995a). *Dissexualität im Lebenslängsschnitt: Theoretische und empirische Untersuchungen zu Phänomenologie und Prognose begutachteter Sexualstraftäter.* Berlin: Springer.

Beier, K. M. (1995b). Aurorismus: Klinische Erscheinungsform einer "weiblichen Analogie" zur Perversion. Geburtsh. *Frauenheilk, 55*(6), 323–330.

Beier, K. M. (1998). Differential typology and prognosis for dissexual behavior—a follow-up study of previously expert-appraised child molesters. *International Journal of Legal Medicine, 111,* 133–141.

Beier, K. M. (2000). Female analogies to perversion. *Journal of Sex and Marital Therapy, 26,* 79–93.

Beier, K. M. (2010). Sexuelle Präferenzstörungen und Bindungsprobleme. *Sexuologie, 17*(1–2), 24–31.

Beier, K. M., & Loewit, K. K. (2004). *Lust in Beziehung. Einführung in die Syndyastische Sexualtherapie.* Berlin: Springer.

Beier, K. M., & Neutze, J. (2009). Das neue "Präventionsprojekt Kinderpornographie" (PPK): Erweiterung des Berliner Ansatzes zur therapeutischen Primärprävention von sexuellem Kindesmissbrauch im Dunkelfeld. *Sexuologie, 16*(1–2), 66–74.

Beier, K. M., Bosinski, H. A. G., & Loewit, K. K. (2005). *Sexualmedizin* (2nd ed.). München: Urban & Fischer.

Beier, K. M., Wille, R., & Wessel, J. (2006). Denial of pregnancy as a reproductive dysfunction: A proposal for international classification systems. *Journal of Psychosomatic Research, 61,* 723–730.

Beier, K. M. (2007). Sexueller Kannibalismus. München, Jena: Elsevier, Urban & Fischer.

Beier, K. M., Neutze, J., Mundt, I. A., et al. (2009). Encouraging self-identified pedophiles and hebephiles to seek professional help: First results of the Berlin prevention project Dunkelfeld (PPD). *Child Abuse & Neglect, 33,* 545–549.

Beitchman, J. H., Zucker, K. J., Hood, J. E., et al. (1991). A review of the short-term effects of child sexual abuse. *Child Abuse & Neglect, 15,* 537–556.

Beitchman, J. H., Zucker, K. J., Hood, J. E., et al. (1992). A review of the long-term effects of child sexual abuse. *Child Abuse & Neglect, 16,* 101–118.

Berglund, H., Lindström, P., & Savic, I. (2006). Brain response to putative pheromones in lesbian women. *Proceedings of the National Academy of Sciences, 103,* 8269–8274.

Blanchard, R. (1989). The concept of autogynephilia and the typology of male gender dysphoria. *Journal of Nervous and Mental Disease, 177,* 616–623.

Blanchard, R., Lykins, A. D., Wherret, D., et al. (2009). Pedophilia, hebephilia, and the DSM-V. *Archives of Sexual Behavior, 38,* 335–350.

Boetticher, A., Nedopil, N., Bosinski, H. A. G., & Saß, H. (2005). Mindestanforderungen für Schuldfähigkeitsgutachten. *Neue Zeitschrift für Strafrecht, 2,* 57–62.

Boetticher, A., Kröber, H. L., Müller-Isberner, R., et al. (2006). Mindestanforderungen für Prognosegutachten. *Neue Zeitschrift für Strafrecht, 10,* 537–544.

Bourke, M. L., & Hernandez, A. E. (2009). The 'Buttner Study' redux: A report of the incidence of hands-on child victimization by child pornography offenders. *Journal of Family Violence, 24,* 183–191.

Bowlby, J. (1969/1973/1980). *Attachment and loss* (Vols. 1, 2, 3). New York: Basic Books.

Braun, M., Wassmer, G., Klotz, T., et al. (2000). Epidemiology of erectile dysfunction: Results of the 'Cologne Male Survey'. *International Journal of Impotence Research, 12,* 305–311.

Bravo,-Dr., Sommer-Studie. Bauer Media Group. (Eds.). (2009). *Liebe, Körper, Sexualität.* München: Forschungsbericht Iconkids & Youth International Research.

Brisch, K. H. (1999). *Bindungsstörungen: Von der Bindungstheorie zur Therapie.* Stuttgart: Klett-Cotta.

Buddeberg, C. (1996). *Sexualberatung. Eine Einführung für Ärzte, Psychotherapeuten und Familienberater* (3rd ed.). Stuttgart: Enke.

Bundesministerium für Familie, Senioren, Frauen und Jugend. (2004). Lebenssituation, Sicherheit und Gesundheit von Frauen in Deutschland. Repräsentative-Studie durchgeführt vom Zentrum für Interdisziplinäre Frauen- und Geschlechterforschung (IFF) der Universität Bielefeld und infas, dem Institut für angewandte Sozialwissenschaft GmbH. einzusehen unter www.bmfsfj.de.

Calvete, E., Orue, I., Estévez, A., Villardón, L., & Padilla, P. (2010). Cyberbullying in adolescents: Modalities and aggressors' profile. *Computers in Human Behavior, 26,* 1128–1135.

Chevret, M., Jaudinot, E., Sullivan, K., et al. (2004). Impact of erectile dysfunction (ED) on sexual life of female partners: Assessment with the index of sexual life (ISL) questionnaire. *Journal of Sexual Medicine, 5,* 595–601.

Chew, K. K., Bremner, A., Jamrozik, K., et al. (2008). Male erectile dysfunction and cardiovascular disease: is there an intimate nexus? *Journal of Sexual Medicine, 5,* 928–934.

Clement, U. (2004). *Systemische Sexualtherapie.* Stuttgart: Klett-Cotta.

Deneke, F. W. (1999). *Psychische Struktur und Gehirn: Die Gestaltung subjektiver Wirklichkeiten.* Stuttgart: Schattauer.

de Vries, A., & Cohen-Kettenis, P. (2012). Clinical management of gender dysphoria in children and adolescents: The dutch approach. *Journal of Homosexuality, 59,* 301–320.

Domes, G., Heinrichs, M., Michel, A., et al. (2007). Oxytocin improves "mind-reading" in humans. *Biological Psychiatry, 61,* 731–733.

Egle, U. T., Hoffmann, S. O., & Steffens, M. (1997). Psychosoziale Risiko- und Schutzfaktoren in Kindheit und Jugend als Prädisposition für psychische Störungen im Erwachsenenalter. *Nervenarzt, 68,* 683–695.

Engelhardt, L., Willers, B., & Pelz, L. (1995). Sexual maturation in East German girls. *Acta Paediatrica, 84,* 1362–1365.

Englert, H., Schaefer, G., Roll, S., et al. (2007). Prevalence of erectile dysfunction among middle-aged men in a metropolitan area in Germany. *International Journal of Impotence Research, 19*(2),183–188.

Feldman, H. A., Goldstein, I., Hatzichristou, D. G., et al. (1994). Impotence and its medical and psychosocial correlates: Results of the Massachusetts male aging study. *Journal of Urology, 151,* 54–61.

Finkelhor, D. (1994). The international epidemiology of child sexual abuse. *Child Abuse & Neglect, 18,* 409–417. doi:10.1016/0145-2134(94)90026-4.

Fisher, W. A., Rosen, R. C., Eardley, I., et al. (2005). Sexual experience of female partners of men with erectile dysfunction: The female experience of men's attitudes to life events and sexuality (females) study. *Journal of Sexual Medicine, 2,* 675–684.

Flaherty, E. G., Thomson, R., Litrownik, A. J., et al. (2009). Adverse childhood exposures and reported child health at age 12. *Academic Pediatrics, 9,* 150–156.

Fraser, L. R., Beyret, E., Milligan, S. R., & Adeoya-Osiguwa, S. A. (2006). Effects of estrogenic xenobiotics on human and mouse spermatozoa. *Human Reproduction, 21,* 1184–1193.

Fröhlich, G. (1998). Psychosomatik männlicher Sexualität. *Sexuologie, 5*(4), 203–211

Gerber, S., Behlia, F., & Hohlfeld, P. (2006). Topical treatment for vulvar vestibulitis with cytokine cream, follow up of a cohort. 6th Congress of the European College for the Study of Vulva Disease, Paris, Sep 21–23 (Abstract).

Görge, G., Flüchter, S., Kirstein, M., & Kunz, T. (2003). Sexualität, erektile Dysfunktion und das Herz: Ein zunehmendes Problem. *Herz, 28,* 284–290.

Grimm, P., & Rhein, S. (2007). *Slapping, Bullying, Snuffing. Zur Problematik von gewalthaltigen und pornografischen Videoclips auf Mobiltelefonen von Jugendlichen.* Berlin: Vistas.

Grimm, P., Rhein, S., & Müller, M. (2010). *Porno im Web 2.0. Die Bedeutung sexualisierter Web-Inhalte in der Lebenswelt von Jugendlichen.* Berlin: Vistas.

Gündel, H., & Stephan, M. (2010). Neurobiologie von Trauma, Traumagedächtnis und Traumafolgen. In J. M. Fegert, U. Ziegenhain, & L. Goldbeck (Eds.), *Traumatisierte Kinder und Jugendliche in Deutschland* (pp. 246–253). Weinheim und München: Juventa.

Hanson, R. K., & Morton-Bourgon, K. (2005). The characteristics of persistent sexual offenders: A meta-analysis of recidivism studies. *Journal of Consulting and Clinical Psychology, 6,* 1154–1163.

Hembree, W. C., Cohen-Kettenis, P., Delemarre-van de Waal, H. A., Gooren, L. J., Meyer, W. J., III, Spack, N. P., Tangpricha, V., & Montori, V. M. (2009). Endocrine treatment of transsexual persons. An endocrine society clinical practice guideline. *Journal of Clinical Endocrinology & Metabolism, 94,* 3132–3154.

Heim, C., Young, L. J., Newport, D. J., Mletzko, T., Miller, A. H., & Nemeroff, C. B. (2009). Lower CSF oxytocin concentrations in women with a history of childhood abuse. *Molecular Psychiatry, 14,* 954–958.

Herkommer, K., Niespodziany, S., Zorn, C., et al. (2006). Versorgung der erektilen Dysfunktion nach radikaler Prostatektomie in Deutschland. *Urologe, 45*(3), 336–342.

Holt-Lunstad, J., Birmingham, W. A., & Light, K. C. (2008). Influence of a "warm touch" support enhancement intervention among married couples on ambulatory blood pressure, oxytocin, alpha amylase, and cortisol. *Psychosomatic medicine, 70,* 976–985.

Humboldt von, W. (1795). Über den Geschlechtsunterschied und dessen Einfluss auf die organische Natur. In F. Schiller (Ed.), *Die Horen* (Vol. 1, 2nd ed., pp. 99–132). Tübingen: Cotta.

Hüther, G. (2005). *Biologie der Angst. Wie aus Stress Gefühle werden* (p. 91). Göttingen: Vandenhoeck.

Hüther, G. (2006). Neurobiologie der Paarbindung. *Sexuologie, 13,* 75–79.

IJzendoorn van, M. H., Huffmeijer, R., Alink, L. R. A., Bakermans-Kranenburg, M. J., & Tops, M. (2011, October). The impact of oxytocin administration on charitable donating is moderated by experience of parental love-withdrawal. *Frontiers in Psychology/Developmental Psychology,* 2(258), 1–8.

Johnson, S., & Zuccarini, D. (2010). Integrating sex and attachment in emotionally focused couple therapy. *Journal of Marital and Family Therapy, 36*(4), 431–445.

Kaufman, J. M., Rosen, R. C., & Mudumbi, R. V. (2009). Treatment benefit of dapoxetine for premature ejaculation: Results from a placebo-controlled phase III trial. *BJU International, 103,* 651–658.

Kendall-Tacket, K. A., Meyer-Williams, L., & Finkelhor, D. (1997). Die Folgen von sexuellem Mißbrauch bei Kindern: Review und Synthese neuerer empirischer Studien. In G. Amann & R. Wipplinger (Eds.), *Sexueller Missbrauch. Überblick zu Forschung, Beratung und Therapie* (pp. 151–186). Tübingen: DGVT.

KIM-Studie. (2008). Kinder + Medien, Computer + Internet. Forschungsbericht Medienpädagogischer Forschungsverbund Südwest (Eds.), (2009), Landesanstalt für Kommunikation. Stuttgart: Baden-Württemberg.

Kinzl, H. (1997). Die Bedeutung der Familienstruktur für die Langzeitfolgen von sexuellem Mißbrauch. In G. Amann & R. Wipplinger (Eds.), *Sexueller Missbrauch Überblick zu Forschung, Beratung und Therapie* (pp. 140–148). Tübingen: DGVT.

Kirsch, P., Esslinger, C., Chen, Q., et al. (2005). Oxytocin modulates neural circuitry for social cognition and fear in humans. *Journal of Neuroscience, 25,* 11489–11493.

Kress D, Loewit K. (2012). Postdoctoral education in Sexual Medicine: The role of modified Balint-groups. *Ärztliche Psychotherapie, 7,* 42–45.

Korte, A., Lehmkuhl, U., Goecker, D., Beier, K. M., Krude, H., & Grueters-Kieslich, A. (2008). Gender identity disorders in childhood and adolescence: Currently debated concepts and treatment strategies. *Deutsches Aerzteblatt International, 105*(48), 834–841.

Landolt, M. A. (2010). Effektivität der Traumatherapie bei Kindern und Jugendlichen. In J. M. Fegert, U. Ziegenhain, & L. Goldbeck (Eds.), *Traumatisierte Kinder und Jugendliche in Deutschland* (S 77–81). Weinheim: Juventa.

Landolt, M. A., & Hensel, T. (Eds.). (2008). *Traumatherapie bei Kindern und Jugendlichen.* Göttingen: Hogrefe.

Langström, N., & Zucker, K. J. (2005). Transvestic fetishism in the general population: Prevalence and correlates. *Journal of Sex & Marital Therapy, 31,* 87–95.

Laumann, E. O., Paik, A., & Rosen, R. C. (1999). Sexual dysfunction in the United States: Prevalence and predictors. *Journal of the American Medical Association, 281,* 537–544.

Laumann, E. O., Nicolosi, A., Glasser, D. B., et al. (2005). Sexual problems among women and men aged 40-80 y: Prevalence and correlates identified in the global study of sexual attitudes and behaviors. *International Journal of Impotence Research, 17,* 39–57.

Leitenberg, H., Greenwald, E., & Tarran, M. J. (1989). The relation between sexual activity among children during preadolescence and/or early adolescence and sexual behavior and sexual adjustment in young adulthood. *Archives of Sexual Behavior, 18,* 299–313.

Loewit, K. K. (1980). The communicative function of human sexuality. A neglected dimension. In R. Forleo & W. Pasini (Eds.), *Medical sexology* (pp. 234–237; 301–318). Littleton: PSG.

Loewit, K. K. (1992). *Die Sprache der Sexualität.* Frankfurt: Fischer.

Loewit, K. K. (2003). Zur Stellung der Sexualmedizin innerhalb der Medizinischen Fächer. *Wiener Medizinische Wochenschrift, 153,* 171–173.

Loewit, K. K. (2005). Sexualmedizin und Balintarbeit. *Sexuologie, 12,* 67–70.

Loewit, K. K., & Beier, K. M. (1998). Standortbestimmung der Sexualmedizin. *Sexuologie, 5,* 49–64.

Lösel, F., & Bliesener, Th. (2003). *Aggression und Delinquenz unter Jugendlichen. Untersuchungen von kognitiven und sozialen Bedingungen.* Neuwied: Luchterhand.

Marcum, C. D. (2007) Interpreting the intentions of internet predators: An examination of online predatory behavior. *Journal of Child Sexual Abuse, 16*(4), 99–114.

Masters, W. H., & Johnson, V. E. (1966). Human sexual response. In Little, Brown & Co., Boston, dt. Ausg (1970) *Die sexuelle Reaktion.* Reinbek: Rowohlt.

Mathers, M. J., Schmitges, J., Klotz, T., & Sommer, F. (2007). Einführung in die Diagnostik und Therapie der Ejakulatio praecox. *Deutsches Arzteblatt, 104*(50), A-3475–A-3480.

McCabe, K. A., & Martin, G. M. (2005) *School violence, the media and criminal justice responses.* New York: Lang.

McCrory, E., De Brito, S. A., & Viding, E. (2011). The impact of childhood maltreatment: A review of neurobiological and genetic factors. *Frontiers in Psychiatry, 2*(48), 1–14.

McMahon, C. G., Park, N. C., Zhao, Y., Rothman, M., & Rivas, D. (2008). Treatment of premature ejaculation (PE) in the Asia-Pacific Region: Results from a phase III doubleblind, parallel-group study of dapoxetine. *Journal of Sexual Medicine, 5*(Suppl. 5), 226–227.

Mendling, W. (2008). Burning Vulva, Vulvodynie, vulväres Vestibulitis-Syndrom. *Frauenarzt, 49*(4), 314–317.

Menesini, E., & Nocentini, A. (2009) Cyberbullying—definition and measurement. *Journal of Psychology, 217*(4), 230–232.

Metz, M. E., & McCarthy, B. W. (2007). The "Good-Enough Sex" model for couple sexual satisfaction. *Sexual and Relationship Therapy, 22*(3), 351–362.

Mitchel, K. J., Finkelhor, D., & Wolak; J. (2001). Risk factors for and impact of online sexual solicitation of youth. *Journal of the American Medical Association, 23*(285), 3011–3014.

Montagu, A. (1987). *Körperkontakt.* Stuttgart: Klett-Cotta.

Montorsi, F. (2005). Prevalence of premature ejaculation: A global and regional perspective. *Journal of Sexual Medicine, 2*(Suppl. 2), 96–102.

Mukamel, R., Ekstrom, A. D., Kaplan, J., Iacoboni, M., & Fried, I. (2010). Single-neuron responses during execution and observation of actions. *Current Biology, 20,* 750–756.

Mullen, P. E. (1997). Der Einfluß von sexuellem Kindesmißbrauch auf die soziale, interpersonelle und sexuelle Funktion im Leben des Erwachsenen und seine Bedeutung in der Entstehung psychischer Probleme. In G. Amann & R. Wipplinger (Eds.), *Sexueller Mißbrauch: Überblick zu Forschung, Beratung und Therapie* (pp. 246–259). Tübingen: DGVT.

Nijs, P. (1997). Zur Behandlung langfristiger Folgen sexuellen Kindesmissbrauchs. *Sexuologie, 4,* 124–131.

Pereda, N., Guilera, G., Forns, M., & Gómez-Benito, J. (2009). The prevalence of child sexual abuse in community and student samples: A meta-analysis. *Clinical Psychology Review, 29,* 328–338. doi:10.1016/j.cpr.2009.02.007.

Pfaff, D. W. (1999). *Drive. Neurobiological and molecular mechanisms of sexual motivation.* Cambridge: MIT.

Ponseti, J., Bosinski, H. A. G., Wolff, S., et al. (2006). A functional endophenotype for sexual orientation in humans. *NeuroImage, 33,* 825–833.

Porst, H., Montorsi, F., Rosen, R. C., et al. (2007). The premature ejaculation Prevalence and attitudes (PEPA) survey: Prevalence, comorbidities, and professional help-seeking. *European Urology, 51,* 816–823.

Rind, B., Tromovitch, P., & Bauserman, R. (1998). A meta-analytic examination of assumed properties of child sexual abuse using college samples. *Psychological Bulletin, 124,* 22–53.

Rosen, R. C., Seidman, S. N., Menza, M. A., et al. (2004). Quality of life, mood, and sexual function: A path analytic model of treatment effects in men with erectile dysfunction and depressive symptoms. *International Journal of Impotence Research, 16,* 334–340.

Rösing, D., & Berberich, H. J. (2004). Krankheits- und behandlungsbedingte Sexualstörungen nach radikaler Prostatektomie—eine bio-psycho-soziale Betrachtung. *Urologe [A], 43*(3), 291–295.

Rösing, D., Klebingat, K. J., Berberich, H. J., et al. (2009). Sexualstörungen des Mannes – Diagnostik und Therapie aus sexualmedizinisch-interdisziplinärer Sicht. *Deutsches Arzteblatt International, 106*(50), 821–828.

Rüegg, J. C. (2003). *Psychosomatik, Psychotherapie und Gehirn: Neuronale Plastizität als Grundlage einer biopsychosozialen Medizin.* Stuttgart: Schattauer.

Rutschky, K., & Wolff, R. (Eds.). (1994). *Handbuch sexueller Mißbrauch.* Hamburg: Klein.

Sabina, Ch., Wolak, J., & Finkelhor, D. (2008). The nature and dynamics of internet pornography exposure for youth. *Cyberpsychology & Behavior, 11*(6), 691–693.

Savic, I., Berglund, H., & Lindström, P. (2005). Brain response to putative pheromones in homosexual men. *Proceedings of the National Academy of Sciences of the United States of America, 102*, 7356–7361.

Schäfer, G. A., Engert, H. S., Ahlers, Ch. J., et al. (2003). Erektionsstörungen und Lebensqualität: Erste Ergebnisse der Berliner Männer-Studie. *Sexuologie, 10*(2/3), 50–60

Schlenker, G. (2004). Östrogene in der Umwelt und damit verbundene Risiken. In E. Wiesner (Ed.), *Handlexikon der tierärztlichen Praxis* (pp. 629vb–629vg). Stuttgart: Enke.

Schnarch, D. M. (1991). *Constructing the sexual crucible*. New York: WW Norton & Co.

Schnarch, D. M. (1997). *Passionate marriage*. New York: WW Norton & Co.

Schurch, B., & Reitz, A. (2004). Botulinumtoxin in der Urologie. *Urologe, 43*, 1410–1415.

Seiwald, J. (1996). *Einfluß von Schwangerschaft und Geburt auf das Sexualleben der Frau*. Dissertation, Med. Fakultät der Universität Innsbruck.

Seto, M. C. (2008). *Pedophilia and sexual off ending against children: Theory, assessment, and intervention*. Washington: American Psychological Association.

Seto, M. C., Cantor, J. M., & Blanchard, R. (2006). Child pornography offenses are a valid diagnostic indicator of pedophilia. *Journal of Abnormal Child Psychology, 115*, 610–615.

Shannon, D. (2008). Online sexual grooming in Sweden—Online and offline sex offences against children as described in Swedish police data. *Journal of Scandinavian Studies in Criminology and Crime Prevention, 9*, 160–180.

Shonkoff, J. P., Boyce, W. T., & McEwen, B. S. (2009). Neuroscience, molecular biology, and the childhood roots of health disparities: Building a new framework for health promotion and disease prevention. *Journal of the American Medical Association, 301*, 2252–2259.

St. Amand, A., Bard, D. E., & Silovsky, J. F. (2008). Meta-analysis of treatment for child sexual behaviour problems: Practice elements and outcomes. *Child Maltreatment, 13*, 145–166.

Steensma, T. D., Biemond, R., de Boer, F., & Cohen-Kettenis, P. T. (2011). Desisting and persisting gender dysphoria after childhood: A qualitative follow-up study. *Clinical Child Psychology and Psychiatry, 16*(4), 499–516.

Stulhofer, A., Busko, V., & Landripet, I. (2010). Pornography, sexual socialization, and satisfaction among young men. *Archives of Sexual Behavior, 39*, 168–178.

Tokunaga, R. S. (2010). Following you home from school: A critical review and synthesis of research on cyberbullying victimization. *Computers in Human Behavior, 26*, 277–287.

Vincent, C. E. (Eds.). (1964). *Human sexuality in medical education and practice*. Springfield: Thomas.

Vogt, H.-J., Loewit, K. K., Wille, R., et al. (1995). Zusatzbezeichnung "Sexualmedizin"—Bedarfsanalyse und Vorschläge für einen Gegenstandskatalog. *Sexuologie, 2*(2), 65–89.

Wagner, M., & Oehlmann, J. (2009). Endocrine disruptors in bottled mineral water: Total estrogenic burden and migration from plastic bottles. *Environmental Science and Pollution Research, 16*, 278 (published online: 10 March 2009).

Wallien, M. S., Swaab, H., & Cohen-Kettenis, P. T. (2007). Psychiatric comorbidity among children with gender identity disorder. *Journal of the American Academy of Child and Adolescent Psychiatry, 46*, 1307–1314.

Watzlawick, P., Beavin, J. H., & Jackson, D. D. (1969). *Menschliche Kommunikation*. Bern: Huber.

Wesiack, W. (1984). *Psychosomatische Medizin in der ärztlichen Praxis*. München: Urban & Schwarzenberg.

Wetzels, P. (1997). Prävalenz sexuellen Kindesmissbrauchs. *Sexuologie, 4*, 89–107.

WHO. (1993). *Internationale Klassifikation psychischer Störungen ICD-10 (Kapitel V (F)) Klinisch-diagnostische Leitlinien*. Bern: Huber

Wickler, W. (1971). *Die Biologie der Zehn Gebote*. München: Piper.

Wickler, W., & Seibt, U. (1984). *Männlich, Weiblich. Der große Unterschied und seine Folgen*. München: Piper.

Willers, B., Engelhardt, L., & Pelz, L. (1996). Sexual maturation in East German boys. *Acta Paediatrica, 85*, 785–788.

Wolak, J., Ybarra, M. L., Mitchell, K., & Finkelhor, D. (2007). Current research knowledge about adolescent victimization via the internet. *Adolescent Medicine, 18,* 325–341.

World Professional Association of Transgender Health (WPATH). (2011). Standards of care. Seventh edition. Retrieved from http//www.wpath.org/.

Zank, S. (1999). Sexualität im Alter. *Sexuologie, 6*(2), 65–87.

Zettl, S., & Hartlapp, J. (1997). *Sexualstörungen durch Krankheit und Therapie. Ein Kompendium für die ärztliche Praxis.* Berlin: Springer.

Index

K. M. Beier, K. K. Loewit, *Sexual Medicine in Clinical Practice,*
DOI 10.1007/978-1-4614-4421-3, © Springer Science+Business Media, LLC 2013